TRIBRID TRAINING

STRENGTH  NA

Published by **www.s** _..uoningcourse.com

www.strengthandconditioningcourse.com

Facebook & Instagram: **@strengthandconditioningcourse**

Cover Image Copyright: Strength and Conditioning Course

Contents

Introduction

Thanks for purchasing a copy of TRIBRID Training.

This book works as both a program with detailed instructions and program cards for each training session, and a logbook with log pages to track your progress.

Over the next 5-pages, there is room for you to fill in some of your personal information, set goals, list your current strengths and weaknesses, and log any injuries or ailments you currently have or are affected by.

From there, we get into the TRIBRID Training!

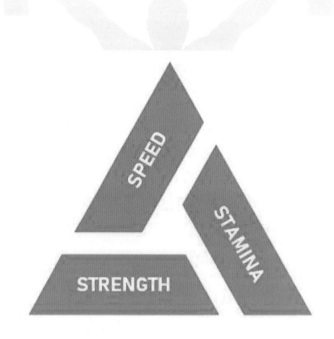

Personal Info

Name:	
Date of Birth:	
Phone:	
Email:	
Date Started:	

Medical Info:	

Weight, Body Fat Percentage and Girth Measurements (Tape Measure)					
Date:					
Weight:					
Body Fat %:					
Neck:					
Chest:					
Arms:					
Forearms:					
Waist:					
Hips:					
Thighs:					
Calves:					

Goals

There are three types of goals:

- **Outcome Goal(s):** The main goal(s) you are working towards and looking to achieve after a set period of time – the main goal is often referred to as the "overarching goal."

- **Performance Goals:** These are benchmarks you are looking to achieve on your way to the main outcome goal.

- **Process Goals:** These are the processes we will take to achieve our outcome goal(s), i.e., I will train 3x a week.

Goals are classed as: (these can be adapted to suit you)

- **Short-Term**: 0-1 Month.

- **Medium-Term**: 1-6 Months.

- **Long-Term:** 6+ Months.

Goals should be SMART:

- Specific.

- Measurable.

- Achievable.

- Relevant.

- Timed.

Short-Term								
Goal:								
Date Set:								
Target Date:								
Achieved:	Y	N	Y	N	Y	N	Y	N

Medium-Term								
Goal:								
Date Set:								
Target Date:								
Achieved:	Y	N	Y	N	Y	N	Y	N

Long-Term								
Goal:								
Date Set:								
Target Date:								
Achieved:	Y	N	Y	N	Y	N	Y	N

Strength and Weaknesses

Strengths + Notes	Weaknesses + Notes

Injury Tracker

Injury	Notes

Key

Here are the key terms and abbreviations used in this program and their meanings:

- Primary Lift = the first strength lift of most importance
- Assistance Lifts = the secondary lifts
- Speed = aim of the session is fast running and sprinting over short distances (high to max effort)
- Tempo = working at a continuous set pace – pushing the pace (high effort)
- Steady State = working at a steady pace (low-moderate effort)
- BB = Barbell
- DB = Dumbbell
- KB = Kettlebell
- MB = Medicine Ball
- ES = Each Side
- ED = Each Direction
- OH = Overhead
- SS1 = Strength Session 1, aka "Primary Press" (named after the main lift)
- SS2 = Strength Session 2, aka "Primary Deadlift" (named after the main lift)
- SS3 = Strength Session 3, aka "Primary Squat" (named after the main lift)
- CS1 = Conditioning Session 1
- CS2 = Conditioning Session 2
- CS3 = Conditioning Session 3
- RPE = Rating of Perceived Exertion
- RIR = Reps in Reserve
- 1RM = 1 Rep Max – most you can lift for 1 repetition
- 5RM = 5 Rep Max – most you can lift for 5 repetitions
- 1RME = 1 Rep Max Estimation, e.g., Multiply your 5RM by 1.15 (add 15%)
- CM = Countermovement – an initial movement in the opposite direction to which you are jumping or throwing
- CMJ = Countermovement Jump (V = Vertical / H = Horizontal)
- CMT = Countermovement Throw
- RDL = Romanian Deadlift
- SLDL = Stiff-Leg Deadlift
- RFESS = Rear Foot Elevated Split Squat (AKA, Bulgarian Split Squat)

Tribrid Training Overview

The aim of Tribrid Training is to make you Strong, Fast and Fit, in a way that is enjoyable and sustainable, albeit gruelling at times – the program is ideal for athletes (some sessions are usually dropped) and those that want to be athletic.

The system works off 3 Quality Strength Training Sessions and 3 Quality Conditioning Sessions a week (you will notice the Tribrid Rule of 3) – a variety of different training splits are explained on the next page.

The 3 strength sessions take place in the gym and centre around free weight training, primarily using the barbell (alternatives are listed + I also have Kettlebell Tribrid).

The 3 conditioning sessions come in the form of running/sprinting (treadmill/road/track) and/or rowing. However, other forms of metabolic conditioning are suggested, such as air bike intervals (you could also add in circuit training).

Although the program recommends an ideal training split throughout the week, this is of course, flexible to accommodate for the busy lifestyles people lead, e.g., both the strength training and conditioning sessions can be completed on the same day.

You can choose to take on all aspects of the program or follow solely the strength program or conditioning program – both programs alone with elicit great results!

Although it is best to stick to the program as strictly as possible, there are some exercise variations and optional/additional exercises and workouts that you can add in or exchange (sprints can be exchanged for the air bike, etc).

All is explained on the program cards. However, if you have any questions about the program at all, drop me an email to: **jay@scc.coach**

Training Splits

Although the Full Tribrid Program works off 6 quality training sessions a week, this can be adapted to suit your specific needs and goals.

You can also choose to reduce the training frequency (how many sessions a week) on your 1st cycle (12-weeks) and progress training frequency on subsequent cycles.

Here are some example splits that build up to the Full Tribrid:

- 1x Strength + 1x Conditioning

- 2x Strength + 1x Conditioning

- 3x Strength + 1x Conditioning

- 1x Strength + 2x Conditioning

- 1x Strength + 3x Conditioning

- 2x Strength + 2x Conditioning

- 2x Strength + 3x Conditioning

- 3x Strength + 2x Conditioning

- 3x Strength + 3x Conditioning – Full Tribrid

If performing 1x Strength session per week, I suggest cycling through SS2 and SS3 on alternating weeks.

If performing 2x Strength sessions per week, cycle through any of the 3 Strength Sessions. However, incorporate SS1 if you want more upper body work.

If performing 1 or 2x Conditioning Sessions per week, I suggest performing the session(s) that best suit your goals or are realistic for the given training week. For example, Steady State and Tempo sessions for more endurance and the Speed session for more speed and power.

Video Tutorials

Video tutorials are available on my YouTube channel: **Coach Jason Curtis**

Here you can find video tutorials for all the strength training exercises, as well as running, plyometric and ballistic training drills that are recommended.

Web: **https://youtube.com/c/coachjasoncurtisacademy**

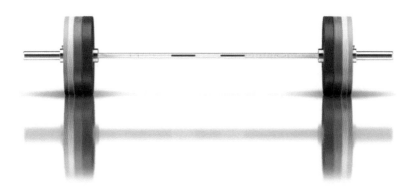

Quantifying Workloads

Tribrid Training uses the RPE Scale (Rating of Perceived Exertion) to quantify training loads. This is done by rating the intensity of an activity from 1-10.

The RPE Scale is a subjective measure, meaning it is based on how you feel (not objective data, i.e., a test score). Therefore, it is not a perfect system and does require some experience to understand what equates to an RPE 7 on various activities or exercises, for example, a 20-min run or 10 reps of a squat. However, it is by far the simplest way to program and monitor training loads.

Note: You can also give an RPE Score for the entire session – over time, this paints a great picture of how you are feeling throughout the training week.

RPE	Intensity
1-2	Very easy
3	Easy
4	Moderate
5-6	Somewhat hard
7-8	Hard
9	Very Hard
10	Maximal

For the primary strength lifts (back squat, bench press, deadlift), once 1RM Maxes have been estimated at week-6 or performed at week-12, percentages of those numbers can be used to quantify training loads.

Just like the RPE Scale, percentages are not a perfect system. However, when applied appropriately, they are a brilliant tool to help optimize progression and keep injuries at bay.

Tribrid Testing

At specific points throughout the program (weeks 6 & 12), testing is carried out to establish baselines, inform programming and ensure the right progressions are being made – **3 Strength Tests** and 3 Conditioning Tests.

Cycle 1:

Test	Week-6 (Score + Date)		Week-12 (Score + Date)	
Back Squat	5RM:		1RM:	
Bench Press	5RM:		1RM:	
Deadlift	5RM:		1RM:	
100m Sprint				
2km Run/Row				
10km Run/Row				

Cycle 2:

Test	Week-6 (Score + Date)		Week-12 (Score + Date)	
Back Squat	5RM:		1RM:	
Bench Press	5RM:		1RM:	
Deadlift	5RM:		1RM:	
100m Sprint				
2km Run/Row				
10km Run/Row				

Test Standards (Male)

The tables on this page and the next show our **Belt System Standards** for both Males and Females split down into 3 different weight categories (some but not all test scores are influenced by the bodyweight categories).

Bodyweight	Belt Standards: Back Squat - Male							
<74kg	40kg	60kg	80kg	100kg	115kg	135kg	150kg	160kg
75-90kg	50kg	70kg	90kg	110kg	125kg	145kg	165kg	185kg
>91kg	60kg	80kg	100kg	120kg	140kg	160kg	180kg	200kg

Bodyweight	Belt Standards: Bench Press - Male							
<74kg	40kg	50kg	60kg	70kg	80kg	90kg	100kg	115kg
75-90kg	45kg	55kg	65kg	75kg	85kg	95kg	110kg	125kg
>91kg	50kg	60kg	70kg	80kg	90kg	100kg	120kg	140kg

Bodyweight	Belt Standards: Deadlift - Male							
<74kg	60kg	80kg	100kg	115kg	130kg	150kg	165kg	180kg
75-90kg	70kg	90kg	110kg	125kg	140kg	160kg	180kg	200kg
>91kg	80kg	100kg	120kg	140kg	165kg	185kg	200kg	230kg

Bodyweight	Belt Standards: 100m Sprint - Male							
<74kg	14.5s	13.5s	13s	12.8s	12.6s	12.4s	12.2s	12s
75-90kg	14.5s	13.5s	13s	12.8s	12.6s	12.4s	12.2s	12s
>91kg	14.5s	13.5s	13s	12.8s	12.6s	12.4s	12.2s	12s

Bodyweight	Belt Standards: 2km Run (Top) / Row (Bottom) - Male							
<74kg	11:15m	10:45m	10:15m	09:30m	08:45m	08:00m	07:00m	06:00m
	09:30m	09:00m	08:30m	08:00m	07:45m	07:15m	06:45m	06:15m
75-90kg	11:30m	11:00m	10:30m	09:45m	09:00m	08:15m	07:15m	06:15m
	09:30m	09:00m	08:30m	08:00m	07:45m	07:15m	06:45m	06:15m
>91kg	12:00m	11:30m	11:00m	10:15m	09:30m	08:45m	07:45m	06:45m
	09:30m	09:00m	08:30m	08:00m	07:45m	07:15m	06:45m	06:15m

Bodyweight	Belt Standards: 10km Run (Top) / Row (Bottom) - Male							
<74kg	68m	63m	58m	54m	50m	46m	42m	38m
	52m	48m	42m	38m	37m	36m	35m	34m
75-90kg	70m	65m	60m	56m	52m	48m	44m	40m
	52m	48m	42m	38m	37m	36m	35m	34m
>91kg	74m	69m	64m	60m	56m	52m	48m	44m
	54m	50m	44m	40m	39m	38m	37m	36m

Test Standards (Female)

Achieve the Black Belt Standard in all 3 Strength Tests to achieve the "**Strength Black Belt**", All 3 Conditioning Tests to achieve the "**Conditioning Black Belt**" and all 6 tests to achieve the "**Tribrid Black Belt**" – the same applies for each colour.

Bodyweight	Belt Standards: Back Squat - Female							
<64kg	25kg	35kg	45kg	55kg	60kg	70kg	80kg	90kg
65-80kg	30kg	40kg	50kg	60kg	70kg	80kg	90kg	100kg
>81kg	35kg	45kg	55kg	65kg	80kg	90kg	100kg	120kg

Bodyweight	Belt Standards: Bench Press - Female							
<64kg	10kg	15kg	20kg	25kg	30kg	35kg	40kg	50kg
65-80kg	15kg	20kg	35kg	30kg	35kg	40kg	45kg	55kg
>81kg	20kg	25kg	30kg	35kg	40kg	45kg	50kg	60kg

Bodyweight	Belt Standards: Deadlift - Female							
<64kg	30kg	40kg	50kg	60kg	70kg	80kg	90kg	100kg
65-80kg	35kg	45kg	55kg	65kg	75kg	90kg	100kg	120kg
>81kg	40kg	50kg	60kg	70kg	85kg	100kg	120kg	140kg

Bodyweight	Belt Standards: 100m Sprint - Female							
<65kg	15.5s	14.5s	14s	13.8s	13.6s	13.4s	13.2s	13s
65-80kg	15.5s	14.5s	14s	13.8s	13.6s	13.4s	13.2s	13s
>81kg	15.5s	14.5s	14s	13.8s	13.6s	13.4s	13.2s	13s

Bodyweight	Belt Standards: 2km Run (Top) / Row (Bottom) - Female							
<64kg	12:45m	11:45m	10:45m	09:45m	09:15m	08:45m	08:15m	07:15m
	10:30m	10:00m	09:30m	09:00m	08:30m	08:00m	07:45m	07:30m
65-80kg	13:00m	12:00m	11:00m	10:00m	09:30m	09:00m	08:30m	07:30m
	10:30m	10:00m	09:30m	09:00m	08:30m	08:00m	07:45m	07:30m
>81kg	13:30m	12:30m	11:30m	10:30m	10:00m	09:30m	09:00m	08:00m
	10:30m	10:00m	09:30m	09:00m	08:30m	08:00m	07:45m	07:30m

Bodyweight	Belt Standards: 10km Run (Top) / Row (Bottom) - Female							
<64kg	72m	68m	62m	58m	54m	50m	46m	42m
	62m	60m	58m	56m	54m	50m	46m	43m
65-80kg	75m	70m	65m	60m	56m	52m	48m	45m
	62m	60m	58m	56m	54m	50m	46m	43m
>81kg	78m	73m	68m	63m	59m	55m	51m	48m
	62m	60m	58m	56m	54m	50m	46m	43m

Tribrid Periodization

The Tribrid Periodization model includes 6 key phases, known as **"The 1st 3"** and **"The 2nd 3"** – the final testing/taper week concludes each 3.

The total length of the model is 12-weeks, and this can be repeated multiple times to cover the span of a training year.

Phase	Duration	Notes
P1 Familiarization	2-Weeks	This phase acts like a preload with moderate levels of volume and intensity – get the muscles working and build familiarity with the exercises (develop technique)
P2 Accumulation	3-Weeks	This phase is about building the base with higher volumes and tempo work on the strength and upping the time/distance of conditioning work
P3 Testing	1-Week	Back Squat – Bench Press – Deadlift – 100m Sprint – 2km Run/Row – 10km Run/Row This week can be a taper if prior to an event
P4 Intensification	3-Weeks	This phase is about upping the intensity (Cluster Sets) and dropping the volume slightly in most areas – volume continues to progress on tempo and steady state conditioning
P5 Realization	2-Weeks	This phase is about peaking for the final test week (or a competition). Intensity increases dramatically (Complex Training) and volume drops significantly
P6 Testing	1-Week	Back Squat – Bench Press – Deadlift – 100m Sprint – 2km Run/Row – 10km Run/Row This week can be a taper if prior to an event

Tribrid Strength Program

The table below gives an overview of the 12-weeks for the primary and main assistance lifts (some rep ranges may differ on specific exercises).

Phase	Week	Primary Lift (Sets/Reps)	Assistance (Sets/Reps)	Advanced Techniques (Primary Lifts Only)
Familiarization	1	3x6	3x8	Lift with a steady tempo
Familiarization	2	3x8	3x10	Lift with a steady tempo
Accumulation	3	3x12	3x12	Tempo: 2 Sec Eccentric
Accumulation	4	3x10	3x12	Tempo: 3 Sec Eccentric
Accumulation	5	3x8	3x12	Tempo: 4 Sec Eccentric
Testing	6	5RMs	3x6	Max out for 5
Intensification	7	3x(2x3)	3x10	Cluster Sets
Intensification	8	3x(3x2)	3x8	Cluster Sets
Intensification	9	3x(2x2)	3x6	Cluster Sets
Realization	10	3x3+3	3x5	Complex Training
Realization	11	3x2+2	3x4	Complex Training
Testing	12	1RMs	3x6	Max out for 1

Note: The advanced training techniques used throughout the program will be fully explained on the relevant program card pages.

During Tribrid Training, we want "3 GOOD SETS" on each lift. This set range maximizes motivation and intent – get your 1st set done, get the 2nd set done and finish with your 3rd – we want every set to be the best it can be!

Tribrid Conditioning Program

The table below gives an overview of the 12-weeks for the conditioning sessions.

Phase	Week	CS1 Run	CS2 Run/Row	CS3 Run/Row
Familiarization	1	20 Min	1 Hour Walk	20 Min
Familiarization	2	4x400m	15 Min	30 Min
Accumulation	3	2x100m + 2x200m + 1x400m + 1x800m = 1800m	2km	5km
Accumulation	4	4x100m + 3x200m + 1x400m + 1x800m = 2200m	3km	6km
Accumulation	5	4x100m + 3x200m + 2x400m + 1x800m = 2600m	5km	8km
Testing	6	100m Sprint	2km Run or Row	10km Run or Row
Intensification	7	4x100m + 3x200m + 2x400m = 1800m	2x3km	6km
Intensification	8	4x100m + 3x200m + 1x400m = 1400m	3x2km	10km
Intensification	9	4x100m + 3x200m = 1000m	2x2km	12km
Realization	10	4x100m + 2x200m = 800m	2x1km	8km
Realization	11	4x100m = 400m	1km	5km
Testing	12	100m Sprint	2km Run or Row	10km Run or Row

Tribrid Strength Warm-Up

The Tribrid warm-up is the same for every strength session. Even the upper body biased session includes bodyweight squats and lunges because movement frequency is key – doing the same warm-up builds familiarity and once the protocol becomes second nature, it makes for an incredibly efficient warm-up.

Plyometrics (jumps) and ballistic exercises (throws) are performed at the end of the warm-up as potentiation. However, these are specifically programmed at the start of each strength session – 1 per session.

In Tribrid Training, we micro-dose (little and often) plyometric and ballistic exercises during the potentiation phase of the warm-up. This protocol raises an individual's arousal levels for the subsequent session, builds reactive strength, power, and tissue resilience over time while reducing the risk of overuse injuries.

Note: Reactive strength is the ability to transition between the eccentric (lengthening) and concentric (shortening) phases of a muscle contraction quickly and forcefully.

Exercise	Sets/Reps/Time	Notes
Run/Row/Ski/Bike	3-6 Mins	RPE 4-5
Bodyweight Squat	1x12	10 Second pause on the last rep (deep squat stretch)
Bodyweight Lunge	1x12	6 Reps with torso rotation and 6 reps with overhead reach
Inchworm Complex	1x5	Crawl out on hands – push-up – downward dog – cobra stretch – downward dog – cobra stretch – return to standing = 1 rep
Arm Circles & Swings	1x10 of Each	10 Arm circles forward – 10 backward – 10 arm swings

Tribrid Conditioning Warm-Up

Low-moderate intensity steady state work does not require a specific warm-up (a brief warm-up is still beneficial). However, I highly recommend raising your heart rate and deep muscle temperature prior to any conditioning session where you are pushing the pace – a 400-500m run or row is usually sufficient.

Prior to any speed or tempo session, I highly recommend you perform a pulse raiser and several running drills to reinforce technique and get your structures primed and ready to go – shake off and get a quick breather between each drill.

Below is my standard pre-track session warm-up, which is ideal for any of the speed sessions in this program – of course, you can tailor it to suit you.

Videos for all the below drills can be found on my **YouTube Channel**

Exercise	Sets/Reps/Time	Notes
Jog	1x200m	RPE 3
High Knees	1x20m	RPE 3-4
Heel Flicks	1x20m	RPE 3-4
Toe Flicks	1x20m	RPE 3-4
High Knee Heel Flicks	1x20m	RPE 5
A-Skips	1x20m	Max Intent
B-Skips	1x20m	Max Intent
Power Skips	1x20m	Max Intent
Bounds	1x20m	Max Intent
Ankle Jumps	1x10	Max Intent

Optional/Additional Work

For the most part, I want you to stick to the program because the volumes and intensities have been programmed to create progressive overload that will maximize performance, build tissue tolerance and minimize the risk of injury – it is NOT just about how you feel on the day, it is about how that training session will affect the rest of the week (self-regulate and know when to reign things in a little).

This being said, time is usually the limiting factor when it comes to including additional work for the core, etc. Therefore, if time and energy allow, you can include the "Optional Work".

Note: **Strength and Conditioning 101 = "What is optimal in the given time and environment"**, which means we want to include the training modes, methods and exercises that pack the most bang for their buck. However, on the flip side, there is a maximum effective dose for any given exercise and therefore, if you do have the time and energy for additional isolation work, you can add it in.

Throughout the program, I will state when a particular exercise is "optional".

Note: BB/DB/Machine calf raises can be added in after any strength session: 3x10. Or perform single-leg calf raises to failure (3 sets on each side).

Here are the core exercises I suggest for the end of any strength or conditioning session: Choose 1-2 exercises – you can also perform 2-3 exercises back-to-back as a Superset (2) or Triset (3).

Exercise	Sets/Reps	Notes
Ab Roll-Out	3x3-10	Increase the intensity by slowing the movement down or pausing at the bottom
GHD Back Extension	3x10-20	Increase the intensity by adding weight
Hanging Knee Raise	3x10-20	Increase the intensity by slowing the movement down
Russian Twist	3x10-20 ES	Increase the intensity by slowing the movement down and/or adding weight
Sit-Up	3x10-20	Increase the intensity by slowing the movement down and/or adding weight

Jot down any additional exercises you might include		
Exercise	**Sets/Reps**	**Notes**

Exercise Variations

Tribrid Training uses a selection of exercises that I deem to have the greatest effects on the movements and muscle groups they are targeting.

Keeping the exercise selection consistent results in the greatest skill progression in the movements and allows us to track progress more effectively.

I highly recommend that you use the programmed exercises for at least 1 full cycle (12-weeks). However, the benefit of mixing exercise selection up is it can make things a little more interesting and can often help you to identify weak points within the chain, e.g., finding a particular muscle struggling during a specific movement.

The table below shows exercise variations for Strength Session 1 (SS1):

Programmed Exercise	Variation 1	Variation 2
BB Bench Press	BB Floor Press	BB Strict/Push Press
Superset: Incline DB Press + DB Bent-Over Row	Superset: High Incline DB Bench Press + DB Incline Bench Row	Superset: Push-Up + BB Inverted Row (Increase reps)
Optional Superset: DB Fly + DB Bent-Over Lateral Raise	Superset: DB Floor Fly + DB Incline Bench Lateral Raise	Superset: Cable Crossover + Cable Horizontal Row/Face Pull
Superset: EZ Biceps Curl + EZ Skull Crusher	Superset: DB Biceps Curl + DB Triceps Extension Superset	Superset: Cable Biceps Curl + Cable Triceps Pushdown

SS1 is the only strength training session to solely concentrate on the upper body. In this session, all the assistance work consists of "Opposing Supersets" that work the pushing and pulling muscles. This style of programming adds more volume while saving time and helps to increase your muscular endurance and work capacity in the gym – take 5-10 seconds rest between the 1st and 2nd exercise within the superset (1-2 deep breaths in and out).

Exercise Variations

The table below shows exercise variations for Strength Session 2 (SS2):

Programmed Exercise	Variation 1	Variation 2
BB Conventional Deadlift	BB Sumo Deadlift	Hex/Trap Bar Deadlift
DB RFESS	DB Split Squat/Alternate Lunge (Forward or Reverse)	DB Walking Lunge
Flat DB Press	DB Floor Press	BB Bench Press (If not performed as the primary lift on SS1)
Single-Arm Row	Cable Single-Arm Row	Suspended Single-Arm Row (increase reps)

The table below shows exercise variations for Strength Session 3 (SS3):

Programmed Exercise	Variation 1	Variation 2
BB Back Squat	BB Front Squat	SSB Squat (Safety Squat Bar)
BB RDL	BB Stiff-Leg Deadlift (from hips)	BB Good Morning
Seated DB Press	Standing DB Press	BB Strict/Push Press (If not performed as the primary lift on SS1)
Pull-Up (Resistance band(s) or weights can be used)	Chin-Up (Resistance band(s) or weights can be used)	Lat Pulldown (Resistance band(s)/machine/cables)

Note: Depending on whether you use a BB bench press or BB overhead (strict/push) press on SS1, you can choose to use the other BB lift on SS2 and SS3 or stick to the DB variations that are programmed.

How to Use the Log Pages

Note: The Program Log pages have been left blank to allow for exercise variations, etc. There is also space to include warm-up/extra sets – the same exercise can continue onto the 2nd row to allow up to 10 sets.

Step 1: Input the date, day, and time.

Step 2: Input your readiness scores – "Good" soreness = no soreness.

Step 3: Input the exercise names.

Step 4: Warm-up appropriately for the training session.

Step 5: Work up to a weight that feels about right for the programmed intensity.

Step 6: Input the weight you lifted in the top box.

Step 7: Input the reps performed (this is programmed on the program card, but you may perform a different number).

Step 8: Input the RPE score for the set – how hard you felt it was out of 10.

Step 9: Input any miscellaneous notes or notes on metabolic conditioning if performed within the strength session.

Step 10: Input the session RPE (score for the whole session).

Note: If conditioning is performed, input notes in the "Conditioning / Notes" section. If performed on a different day to the strength session, input the date of the conditioning session in the box to start – readiness scores for both strength and conditioning sessions can be completed separately (see example).

See an example on the following page.

Program Log Example: Date: ____ / ____ / ____ Day: _____ Time: _____

Exercise	Set 1		Set 2		Set 3		Set 4		Set 5	
	WEIGHT		*WEIGHT*		*WEIGHT*		*WEIGHT*		*WEIGHT*	
	REP	*RPE*	*REP*	*RPE*	*REP*	*RPE*	*REP*	*RPE*	*REP*	*RPE*
EXAMPLE	120		120							
	10	7	10	8						

Conditioning / Notes	Readiness	Bad	Ok	Good
Input the date of the conditioning session if different to the strength session and fill out the readiness scores for each training session separately: Denote an "S" for Strength and a "C" for Conditioning – see the soreness box for an example.	Sleep:		✓	
	Energy:			✓
	Mood:			✓
	Soreness:	S	C	

Session RPE: _____

Tribrid Program Card 1

Phase 1: Familiarization – Week-1

Strength Session 1: Primary Press

Suggested Day: Monday

Aim to be on your working sets on the primary lift within 3-4 warm-up sets. On Assistance lifts, you can perform 1-2 warm-up sets to groove the movements (if needed). However, on all exercises, we want **"3 GOOD SETS"**.

Exercise	Sets/Reps	Intensity	Rest	Notes
Optional: MB CM Chest Throw	5x1	Max Intent	5-10 Secs	Or Overhead (OH) CM Throw if doing a Strict/Push Press / Use a 3-5kg MB
BB Bench Press	3x6	RPE 6	2 Mins	Work on technique
Superset: Incline DB Press + DB Bent-Over Row	3x8+8	RPE 6	1-2 Mins	Take 5-10 seconds rest between the two exercises – 1-2 deep breaths
Optional Superset: DB Fly + DB Bent-Over Lateral Raise	3x8+8	RPE 6	1-2 Mins	Include this superset if you have the time and energy
Superset: EZ Biceps Curl + EZ Skull Crusher	3x8+8	RPE 6	1-2 Mins	Take 5-10 seconds rest between the two exercises – 1-2 deep breaths
		RPE 6	10-30 Secs	Optional Core: Your choice from page-24

Conditioning Session 1: Steady State (CS1 progresses to be the speed session)

Suggested Day: Tuesday

Activity	Description
Run (Steady State)	20 Minute Run: Steady Pace – RPE 3 Don't aim for any particular distance. Just run for 20 mins

Alternative: 5x30 Secs Work, 30 Secs Rest (RPE 8) on a cardio machine (rower, bike, etc), or on equipment such as battle ropes, slam balls or the prowler, etc (post SS1 or another time).

Date: ____ / ____ / ____   Day: _____   Time: _____

Exercise	Set 1		Set 2		Set 3		Set 4		Set 5	
	WEIGHT		WEIGHT		WEIGHT		WEIGHT		WEIGHT	
	REP	RPE	REP	RPE	REP	RPE	REP	RPE	REP	RPE

Conditioning / Notes	Readiness	Bad	Ok	Good
	Sleep:			
	Energy:			
	Mood:			
	Soreness:			

Session RPE: _____

Tribrid Program Card 2

Phase 1: Familiarization – Week-1

Strength Session 2: Primary Deadlift

Suggested Day: Wednesday

Aim to be on your working sets on the primary lift within 3-4 warm-up sets. On Assistance lifts, you can perform 1-2 warm-up sets to groove the movements (if needed). However, on all exercises, we want **"3 GOOD SETS"**.

Exercise	Sets/Reps	Intensity	Rest	Notes
Optional: HCMJ	5x1	Max Intent	5-10 Secs	Horizontal (Broad) Countermovement Jump
BB Conventional Deadlift	3x6	RPE 6	2 Mins	Work on technique
DB RFESS	3x8 ES	RPE 6	1-2 Mins	Work on technique
Flat DB Press	3x8	RPE 6	1-2 Mins	Work on technique
Single-Arm Row	3x8 ES	RPE 6	1-2 Mins	Work on technique
		RPE 6	10-30 Secs	Optional Core: Your choice from page-24

Conditioning Session 2: Walk (CS2 progresses to be a tempo session)

Suggested Day: Thursday

Activity	Description
Walk	1 Hour Recovery Walk – RPE 1-3

Alternative: 30–60 Min steady state work (RPE 2-3) on a cardio machine.

Program Log 2:   Date: ____ / ____ / ____   Day: _____   Time: _____

Exercise	Set 1		Set 2		Set 3		Set 4		Set 5	
	WEIGHT		WEIGHT		WEIGHT		WEIGHT		WEIGHT	
	REP	RPE	REP	RPE	REP	RPE	REP	RPE	REP	RPE

Conditioning / Notes	Readiness	Bad	Ok	Good
	Sleep:			
	Energy:			
	Mood:			
	Soreness:			

Session RPE: _____

Tribrid Program Card 3

Phase 1: Familiarization – Week-1

Strength Session 3: Primary Squat

Suggested Day: Friday

Aim to be on your working sets on the primary lift within 3-4 warm-up sets. On Assistance lifts, you can perform 1-2 warm-up sets to groove the movements (if needed). However, on all exercises, we want **"3 GOOD SETS"**.

Exercise	Sets/Reps	Intensity	Rest	Notes
Optional: VCMJ	5x1	Max Intent	5-10 Secs	Vertical Countermovement Jump
BB Back Squat	3x6	RPE 6	2 Mins	Work on technique
BB RDL	3x8	RPE 6	1-2 Mins	Work on technique
Seated DB Press	3x8	RPE 6	1-2 Mins	Work on technique
Pull-Up	3xMax	RPE 9-10	1-2 Mins	Resistance band(s) can be used to regress the movement or weight can be added to progress it – aim for a min of 2 reps and a max of 10 if using bands
		RPE 6	10-30 Secs	Optional Core: Your choice from page-24

Conditioning Session 3: Steady State (CS3 is the steady state session)

Suggested Day: Saturday/Sunday

Activity	Description
Run/Row (Steady State)	20 Minute Run/Row: Steady Pace – RPE 3 Don't aim for any particular distance. Just run for 20 mins

Alternative: 5x30 Secs Work, 30 Secs Rest (RPE 8) on a cardio machine (rower, bike, etc), or

on equipment such as battle ropes, slam balls or the prowler, etc (post SS3 or another time).

Program Log 3:   Date: ____ / ____ / ____ Day: _____ Time: _____

Exercise	Set 1 WEIGHT		Set 2 WEIGHT		Set 3 WEIGHT		Set 4 WEIGHT		Set 5 WEIGHT	
	REP	RPE	REP	RPE	REP	RPE	REP	RPE	REP	RPE

Conditioning / Notes	Readiness	Bad	Ok	Good
	Sleep:			
	Energy:			
	Mood:			
	Soreness:			

Session RPE: _____

35

Tribrid Program Card 4

Phase 1: Familiarization – Week-2

Strength Session 1: Primary Press

Suggested Day: Monday

Aim to be on your working sets on the primary lift within 3-4 warm-up sets. On Assistance lifts, you can perform 1-2 warm-up sets to groove the movements (if needed). However, on all exercises, we want **"3 GOOD SETS"**.

Exercise	Sets/Reps	Intensity	Rest	Notes
Optional: MB CM Chest Throw	5x1	Max Intent	5-10 Secs	Or Overhead (OH) CM Throw if doing a Strict/Push Press / Use a 3-5kg MB
BB Bench Press	3x8	RPE 6	2 Mins	Work on technique
Superset: Incline DB Press + DB Bent-Over Row	3x10+10	RPE 6	1-2 Mins	Take 5-10 seconds rest between the two exercises – 1-2 deep breaths
Optional Superset: DB Fly + DB Bent-Over Lateral Raise	3x10+10	RPE 6	1-2 Mins	Include this superset if you have the time and energy
Superset: EZ Biceps Curl + EZ Skull Crusher	3x10+10	RPE 6	1-2 Mins	Take 5-10 seconds rest between the two exercises – 1-2 deep breaths
		RPE 6	10-30 Secs	Optional Core: Your choice from page-24

Conditioning Session 1: Speed

Suggested Day: Tuesday

Activity	Description	Rest
Run (Speed)	1x400m – RPE 4	3 Mins
	1x400m – RPE 5	3 Mins
	1x400m – RPE 6-7	3 Mins
	1x400m – RPE 7	N/A
Total Distance	1600m	N/A

Alternative: Perform distances on a rower or ski ERG or divide the distances by 10 and perform them as calories on an air bike (RPE 8) – follow the same rest periods (half them if on the air bike).

Program Log 4:   Date: ____ / ____ / ____   Day: _____   Time: _____

Exercise	Set 1		Set 2		Set 3		Set 4		Set 5	
	WEIGHT		WEIGHT		WEIGHT		WEIGHT		WEIGHT	
	REP	RPE	REP	RPE	REP	RPE	REP	RPE	REP	RPE

Conditioning / Notes	Readiness	Bad	Ok	Good
	Sleep:			
	Energy:			
	Mood:			
	Soreness:			

Session RPE: _____

Tribrid Program Card 5

Phase 1: Familiarization – Week-2

Strength Session 2: Primary Deadlift

Suggested Day: Wednesday

Aim to be on your working sets on the primary lift within 3-4 warm-up sets. On Assistance lifts, you can perform 1-2 warm-up sets to groove the movements (if needed). However, on all exercises, we want **"3 GOOD SETS"**.

Exercise	Sets/Reps	Intensity	Rest	Notes
Optional: HCMJ	5x1	Max Intent	5-10 Secs	Horizontal (Broad) Countermovement Jump
BB Conventional Deadlift	3x8	RPE 6	2 Mins	Work on technique
DB RFESS	3x10 ES	RPE 6	1-2 Mins	Work on technique
Flat DB Press	3x10	RPE 6	1-2 Mins	Work on technique
Single-Arm Row	3x10 ES	RPE 6	1-2 Mins	Work on technique
		RPE 6	10-30 Secs	Optional Core: Your choice from page-24

Conditioning Session 2: Tempo

Suggested Day: Thursday

Activity	Description
Run/Row (Tempo)	15 Minute Run/Row – RPE 4-5 (Push the pace a little) Don't aim for any particular distance. Just run for 15 mins

Alternative: Perform 6x30 Secs Work, 30 Secs Rest (RPE 8) on a cardio machine (rower, bike, etc), or on equipment such as battle ropes, slam balls or the prowler, etc (post SS2 or another time).

Program Log 5:   Date: ____ / ____ / ____   Day: _____   Time: _____

Exercise	Set 1		Set 2		Set 3		Set 4		Set 5	
	WEIGHT		*WEIGHT*		*WEIGHT*		*WEIGHT*		*WEIGHT*	
	REP	*RPE*	*REP*	*RPE*	*REP*	*RPE*	*REP*	*RPE*	*REP*	*RPE*

Conditioning / Notes	Readiness	Bad	Ok	Good
	Sleep:			
	Energy:			
	Mood:			
	Soreness:			

Session RPE: _____

Tribrid Program Card 6

Phase 1: Familiarization – Week-2

Strength Session 3: Primary Squat

Suggested Day: Friday

Aim to be on your working sets on the primary lift within 3-4 warm-up sets. On Assistance lifts, you can perform 1-2 warm-up sets to groove the movements (if needed). However, on all exercises, we want **"3 GOOD SETS"**.

Exercise	Sets/Reps	Intensity	Rest	Notes
Optional: VCMJ	5x1	Max Intent	5-10 Secs	Vertical Countermovement Jump
BB Back Squat	3x8	RPE 6	2 Mins	Work on technique
BB RDL	3x10	RPE 6	1-2 Mins	Work on technique
Seated DB Press	3x10	RPE 6	1-2 Mins	Work on technique
Pull-Up	3xMax	RPE 9-10	1-2 Mins	Resistance band(s) can be used to regress the movement or weight can be added to progress it – aim for a min of 2 reps and a max of 10 if using bands
		RPE 6	10-30 Secs	Optional Core: Your choice from page-24

Conditioning Session 3: Steady State

Suggested Day: Saturday/Sunday

Activity	Description
Run/Row (Steady State)	30 Minute Run/Row: Steady Pace – RPE 3 Don't aim for any particular distance. Just run for 20 mins

Alternative: Perform 6x30 Secs Work, 30 Secs Rest (RPE 8) on a cardio machine (rower, bike, etc), or on equipment such as battle ropes, slam balls or the prowler, etc (post SS3 or another time).

Exercise	Set 1		Set 2		Set 3		Set 4		Set 5	
	WEIGHT		*WEIGHT*		*WEIGHT*		*WEIGHT*		*WEIGHT*	
	REP	*RPE*	*REP*	*RPE*	*REP*	*RPE*	*REP*	*RPE*	*REP*	*RPE*

Conditioning / Notes	Readiness	Bad	Ok	Good
	Sleep:			
	Energy:			
	Mood:			
	Soreness:			

Session RPE: _____

Tribrid Program Card 7

Phase 2: Accumulation – Week-1 (Week-3 of the program)

Strength Session 1: Primary Press

Tempo is written with 4 numbers (the first being the first movement), for example:

Back Squat & Bench Press: 21X2 = 2 seconds down (eccentric), 1 second pause at the bottom, fast as you can up (concentric), 2 second reset at the top.

Deadlift: X122 = fast as you can up (concentric), 1 second pause at the top, 2 seconds down (eccentric), 2 second reset at the bottom.

Exercise	Sets/Reps	Intensity	Rest	Notes
Optional: MB CM Chest Throw	5x1	Max Intent	5-10 Secs	Or Overhead (OH) CM Throw if doing a Strict/Push Press / Use a 3-5kg MB
BB Bench Press	3x12	RPE 7	2 Mins	**Tempo: 21X2**
Superset: Incline DB Press + DB Bent-Over Row	3x12+12	RPE 6-7	1-2 Mins	Take 5-10 seconds rest between the two exercises – 1-2 deep breaths
Optional Superset: DB Fly + DB Bent-Over Lateral Raise	3x12+12	RPE 6-7	1-2 Mins	Include this superset if you have the time and energy
Superset: EZ Biceps Curl + EZ Skull Crusher	3x12+12	RPE 6-7	1-2 Mins	Take 5-10 seconds rest between the two exercises – 1-2 deep breaths
		RPE 6-7	10-30 Secs	Optional Core: Your choice from page-24

Conditioning Session 1: Speed (rest = between sets or the next distance).

Activity	Description	Rest
Run (Speed)	2x100m – 1st RPE 6 / 2nd RPE 8	2 Mins
	2x200m – RPE 6-7	2 Mins
	1x400m – RPE 6-7	2 Mins
	1x800m – RPE 7	N/A
Total Distance	1800m	N/A

Alternative: Perform distances on a rower or ski ERG or divide the distances by 10 and perform them as calories on an air bike (RPE 8) – follow the same rest periods (half them if on the air bike).

Program Log 7:   Date: ____ / ____ / ____ Day: _____ Time: _____

Exercise	Set 1 WEIGHT		Set 2 WEIGHT		Set 3 WEIGHT		Set 4 WEIGHT		Set 5 WEIGHT	
	REP	RPE	REP	RPE	REP	RPE	REP	RPE	REP	RPE

Conditioning / Notes	Readiness	Bad	Ok	Good
	Sleep:			
	Energy:			
	Mood:			
	Soreness:			

Session RPE: _____

Tribrid Program Card 8

Phase 2: Accumulation – Week-1 (Week-3 of the program)

Strength Session 2: Primary Deadlift

Deadlift Tempo Example: X122 = fast as you can up (concentric), 1 second pause at the top, 2 seconds down (eccentric), 2 second reset at the bottom.

Exercise	Sets/Reps	Intensity	Rest	Notes
Optional: HCMJ	3x2	Max Intent	5-10 Secs	Horizontal (Broad) Countermovement Jump
BB Conventional Deadlift	3x12	RPE 7	2 Mins	**Tempo: X122**
DB RFESS	3x12 ES	RPE 6-7	1-2 Mins	Work at a steady tempo
Flat DB Press	3x12	RPE 6-7	1-2 Mins	Work at a steady tempo
Single-Arm Row	3x12 ES	RPE 6-7	1-2 Mins	Work at a steady tempo
		RPE 6-7	10-30 Secs	Optional Core: Your choice from page-24

Conditioning Session 2: Tempo

Activity	Description
Run/Row (Tempo)	2km Run/Row – RPE 5-6 (Push the pace a little)

Alternative: Perform 8x45 Secs Work, 15 Secs Rest (RPE 8) on a cardio machine (rower, bike, etc), or on equipment such as battle ropes, slam balls or the prowler, etc (post SS2 or another time).

Program Log 8:   Date: ____ / ____ / ____ Day: _____ Time: _____

Exercise	Set 1 WEIGHT		Set 2 WEIGHT		Set 3 WEIGHT		Set 4 WEIGHT		Set 5 WEIGHT	
	REP	RPE	REP	RPE	REP	RPE	REP	RPE	REP	RPE

Conditioning / Notes	Readiness	Bad	Ok	Good
	Sleep:			
	Energy:			
	Mood:			
	Soreness:			

Session RPE: _____

Tribrid Program Card 9

Phase 2: Accumulation – Week-1 (Week-3 of the program)

Strength Session 3: Primary Squat

Back Squat Tempo Example: 21X2 = 2 seconds down (eccentric), 1 second pause at the bottom, fast as you can up (concentric), 2 second reset at the top.

Exercise	Sets/Reps	Intensity	Rest	Notes
Optional: VCMJ	3x2	Max Intent	5-10 Secs	Vertical Countermovement Jump
BB Back Squat	3x12	RPE 7	2 Mins	**Tempo: 21X2**
BB RDL	3x12	RPE 6-7	1-2 Mins	Work at a steady tempo
Seated DB Press	3x12	RPE 6-7	1-2 Mins	Work at a steady tempo
Pull-Up	3xMax	RPE 9-10	1-2 Mins	Resistance band(s) can be used to regress the movement or weight can be added to progress it – aim for a min of 2 reps and a max of 10 if using bands
		RPE 6	10-30 Secs	Optional Core: Your choice from page-24

Conditioning Session 3: Steady State

Activity	Description
Run/Row (Steady State)	5km Run/Row – RPE 3-4

Alternative: Perform 8x45 Secs Work, 15 Secs Rest (RPE 8) on a cardio machine (rower, bike, etc), or on equipment such as battle ropes, slam balls or the prowler, etc (post SS3 or another time).

Program Log 9:   Date: ____ / ____ / ____ Day: _____ Time: _____

Exercise	Set 1 WEIGHT		Set 2 WEIGHT		Set 3 WEIGHT		Set 4 WEIGHT		Set 5 WEIGHT	
	REP	RPE	REP	RPE	REP	RPE	REP	RPE	REP	RPE

Conditioning / Notes	Readiness	Bad	Ok	Good
	Sleep:			
	Energy:			
	Mood:			
	Soreness:			

Session RPE: _____

Tribrid Program Card 10

Phase 2: Accumulation – Week-2 (Week-4 of the program)

Strength Session 1: Primary Press

Bench Press Tempo Example: 31X2 = 3 seconds down (eccentric), 1 second pause at the bottom, fast as you can up (concentric), 2 second reset at the top.

Exercise	Sets/Reps	Intensity	Rest	Notes
Optional: MB CM Chest Throw	5x1	Max Intent	5-10 Secs	Or Overhead (OH) CM Throw if doing a Strict/Push Press / Use a 3-5kg MB
BB Bench Press	3x10	RPE 7-8	2 Mins	**Tempo:** 31X2
Superset: Incline DB Press + DB Bent-Over Row	3x12+12	RPE 6-7	1-2 Mins	Take 5-10 seconds rest between the two exercises – 1-2 deep breaths
Optional Superset: DB Fly + DB Bent-Over Lateral Raise	3x12+12	RPE 6-7	1-2 Mins	Include this superset if you have the time and energy
Superset: EZ Biceps Curl + EZ Skull Crusher	3x12+12	RPE 6-7	1-2 Mins	Take 5-10 seconds rest between the two exercises – 1-2 deep breaths
		RPE 6-7	10-30 Secs	Optional Core: Your choice from page-24

Conditioning Session 1: Speed (rest = between sets or the next distance).

Activity	Description	Rest
Run (Speed)	4x100m – 1st RPE 6 / 2nd RPE 8 / 3rd RPE 9 / 4th RPE 10	2 Mins
	3x200m – RPE 8	2 Mins
	1x400m – RPE 7	2 Mins
	1x800m – RPE 7	N/A
Total Distance	2200m	N/A

Alternative: Perform distances on a rower or ski ERG or divide the distances by 10 and perform them as calories on an air bike (RPE 8) – follow the same rest periods (half them if on the air bike).

Program Log 10:   Date: ____ / ____ / ____   Day: _____   Time: _____

Exercise	Set 1		Set 2		Set 3		Set 4		Set 5	
	WEIGHT		*WEIGHT*		*WEIGHT*		*WEIGHT*		*WEIGHT*	
	REP	*RPE*	*REP*	*RPE*	*REP*	*RPE*	*REP*	*RPE*	*REP*	*RPE*

Conditioning / Notes	Readiness	Bad	Ok	Good
	Sleep:			
	Energy:			
	Mood:			
	Soreness:			

Session RPE: _____

49

Tribrid Program Card 11

Phase 2: Accumulation – Week-2 (Week-4 of the program)

Strength Session 2: Primary Deadlift

Deadlift Tempo Example: X132 = fast as you can up (concentric), 1 second pause at the top, 3 seconds down (eccentric), 2 second reset at the bottom.

Exercise	Sets/Reps	Intensity	Rest	Notes
Optional: HCMJ	3x2	Max Intent	5-10 Secs	Horizontal (Broad) Countermovement Jump
BB Conventional Deadlift	3x10	RPE 7-8	2 Mins	**Tempo: X132**
DB RFESS	3x12 ES	RPE 6-7	1-2 Mins	Work at a steady tempo
Flat DB Press	3x12	RPE 6-7	1-2 Mins	Work at a steady tempo
Single-Arm Row	3x12 ES	RPE 6-7	1-2 Mins	Work at a steady tempo
		RPE 6-7	10-30 Secs	Optional Core: Your choice from page-24

Conditioning Session 2: Tempo

Activity	Description
Run/Row (Tempo)	3km Run/Row – RPE 6-7 (Push the pace a little)

Alternative: Perform 8x60 Secs Work, 20 Secs Rest (RPE 8) on a cardio machine (rower, bike, etc), or on equipment such as battle ropes, slam balls or the prowler, etc (post SS2 or another time).

50

Program Log 11:   Date: ____ / ____ / ____ Day: _____ Time: _____

Exercise	Set 1 WEIGHT		Set 2 WEIGHT		Set 3 WEIGHT		Set 4 WEIGHT		Set 5 WEIGHT	
	REP	RPE	REP	RPE	REP	RPE	REP	RPE	REP	RPE

Conditioning / Notes	Readiness	Bad	Ok	Good
	Sleep:			
	Energy:			
	Mood:			
	Soreness:			

Session RPE: _____

Tribrid Program Card 12

Phase 2: Accumulation – Week-2 (Week-4 of the program)

Strength Session 3: Primary Squat

Squat Tempo Example: 31X2 = 3 seconds down (eccentric), 1 second pause at the bottom, fast as you can up (concentric), 2 second reset at the top.

Exercise	Sets/Reps	Intensity	Rest	Notes
Optional: VCMJ	3x2	Max Intent	5-10 Secs	Vertical Countermovement Jump
BB Back Squat	3x10	RPE 7-8	2 Mins	**Tempo: 31X2**
BB RDL	3x12	RPE 6-7	1-2 Mins	Work at a steady tempo
Seated DB Press	3x12	RPE 6-7	1-2 Mins	Work at a steady tempo
Pull-Up	3xMax	RPE 9-10	1-2 Mins	Resistance band(s) can be used to regress the movement or weight can be added to progress it – aim for a min of 2 reps and a max of 10 if using bands
		RPE 6	10-30 Secs	Optional Core: Your choice from page-24

Conditioning Session 3: Steady State

Activity	Description
Run/Row (Steady State)	6km Run/Row – RPE 3-4

Alternative: Perform 8x60 Secs Work, 20 Secs Rest (RPE 8) on a cardio machine (rower, bike, etc), or on equipment such as battle ropes, slam balls or the prowler, etc (post SS3 or another time).

Program Log 12:   Date: ____ / ____ / ____   Day: _____   Time: _____

Exercise	Set 1		Set 2		Set 3		Set 4		Set 5	
	WEIGHT		WEIGHT		WEIGHT		WEIGHT		WEIGHT	
	REP	RPE	REP	RPE	REP	RPE	REP	RPE	REP	RPE

Conditioning / Notes	Readiness	Bad	Ok	Good
	Sleep:			
	Energy:			
	Mood:			
	Soreness:			

Session RPE: _____

Tribrid Program Card 13

Phase 2: Accumulation – Week-3 (Week-5 of the program)

Strength Session 1: Primary Press

Bench Press Tempo Example: 41X2 = 4 seconds down (eccentric), 1 second pause at the bottom, fast as you can up (concentric), 2 second reset at the top.

Exercise	Sets/Reps	Intensity	Rest	Notes
Optional: MB CM Chest Throw	5x1	Max Intent	5-10 Secs	Or Overhead (OH) CM Throw if doing a Strict/Push Press / Use a 3-5kg MB
BB Bench Press	3x8	RPE 7-8	2-3 Mins	**Tempo: 41X2**
Superset: Incline DB Press + DB Bent-Over Row	3x12+12	RPE 6-7	1-2 Mins	Take 5-10 seconds rest between the two exercises – 1-2 deep breaths
Optional Superset: DB Fly + DB Bent-Over Lateral Raise	3x12+12	RPE 6-7	1-2 Mins	Include this superset if you have the time and energy
Superset: EZ Biceps Curl + EZ Skull Crusher	3x12+12	RPE 6-7	1-2 Mins	Take 5-10 seconds rest between the two exercises – 1-2 deep breaths
		RPE 6-7	10-30 Secs	Optional Core: Your choice from page-24

Conditioning Session 1: Speed (rest = between sets or the next distance).

Activity	Description	Rest
Run (Speed)	4x100m – 1st RPE 6 / 2nd RPE 8 / 3rd RPE 9 / 4th RPE 10	2 Mins
	3x200m – RPE 8	2 Mins
	2x400m – RPE 7	2 Mins
	1x800m – RPE 7	N/A
Total Distance	2600m	N/A

Alternative: Perform distances on a rower or ski ERG or divide the distances by 10 and perform them as calories on an air bike (RPE 8) – follow the same rest periods (half them if on the air bike).

Exercise	Set 1		Set 2		Set 3		Set 4		Set 5	
	WEIGHT		WEIGHT		WEIGHT		WEIGHT		WEIGHT	
	REP	RPE	REP	RPE	REP	RPE	REP	RPE	REP	RPE

Conditioning / Notes	Readiness	Bad	Ok	Good
	Sleep:			
	Energy:			
	Mood:			
	Soreness:			

Session RPE: _____

Tribrid Program Card 14

Phase 2: Accumulation – Week-2 (Week-5 of the program)

Strength Session 2: Primary Deadlift

Deadlift Tempo Example: X142 = fast as you can up (concentric), 1 second pause at the top, 4 seconds down (eccentric), 2 second reset at the bottom.

Exercise	Sets/Reps	Intensity	Rest	Notes
Optional: HCMJ	3x3	Max Intent	10-15 Secs	Horizontal (Broad) Countermovement Jump
BB Conventional Deadlift	3x8	RPE 7-8	2-3 Mins	**Tempo: X142**
DB RFESS	3x12 ES	RPE 6-7	1-2 Mins	Work at a steady tempo
Flat DB Press	3x12	RPE 6-7	1-2 Mins	Work at a steady tempo
Single-Arm Row	3x12 ES	RPE 6-7	1-2 Mins	Work at a steady tempo
		RPE 6-7	10-30 Secs	Optional Core: Your choice from page-24

Conditioning Session 2: Tempo

Activity	Description
Run/Row (Tempo)	5km Run/Row – RPE 6-7 (Push the pace a little)

Alternative: Perform 6x90 Secs Work, 30 Secs Rest (RPE 8) on a cardio machine (rower, bike, etc), or on equipment such as battle ropes, slam balls or the prowler, etc (post SS2 or another time).

Program Log 14: Date: ____ / ____ / ____ Day: _____ Time: _____

Exercise	Set 1 WEIGHT		Set 2 WEIGHT		Set 3 WEIGHT		Set 4 WEIGHT		Set 5 WEIGHT	
	REP	RPE	REP	RPE	REP	RPE	REP	RPE	REP	RPE

Conditioning / Notes	Readiness	Bad	Ok	Good
	Sleep:			
	Energy:			
	Mood:			
	Soreness:			

Session RPE: _____

Tribrid Program Card 15

Phase 2: Accumulation – Week-2 (Week-5 of the program)

Strength Session 3: Primary Squat

Squat Tempo Example: 41X2 = 4 seconds down (eccentric), 1 second pause at the bottom, fast as you can up (concentric), 2 second reset at the top.

Exercise	Sets/Reps	Intensity	Rest	Notes
Optional: VCMJ	3x3	Max Intent	10-15 Secs	Vertical Countermovement Jump
BB Back Squat	3x8	RPE 7-8	2-3 Mins	**Tempo: 41X2**
BB RDL	3x12	RPE 6-7	1-2 Mins	Work at a steady tempo
Seated DB Press	3x12	RPE 6-7	1-2 Mins	Work at a steady tempo
Pull-Up	3xMax	RPE 9-10	1-2 Mins	Resistance band(s) can be used to regress the movement or weight can be added to progress it – aim for a min of 2 reps and a max of 10 if using bands
		RPE 6	10-30 Secs	Optional Core: Your choice from page-24

Conditioning Session 3: Steady State

Activity	Description
Run/Row (Steady State)	8km Run/Row – RPE 3-4

Alternative: Perform 6x90 Secs Work, 30 Secs Rest (RPE 8) on a cardio machine (rower, bike, etc), or on equipment such as battle ropes, slam balls or the prowler, etc (post SS3 or another time).

Date: ____ / ____ / ____   Day: _____   Time: _____

Exercise	Set 1 WEIGHT		Set 2 WEIGHT		Set 3 WEIGHT		Set 4 WEIGHT		Set 5 WEIGHT	
	REP	RPE	REP	RPE	REP	RPE	REP	RPE	REP	RPE

Conditioning / Notes	Readiness	Bad	Ok	Good
	Sleep:			
	Energy:			
	Mood:			
	Soreness:			

Session RPE: _____

Week-6 Testing/Taper

During 6-week testing, there are 6 tests to complete.

1. 5RM Back Squat
2. 5RM Bench Press
3. 5RM Deadlift
4. 100m Sprint
5. 2km Run or Row
6. 10km Run or Row

I suggest completing the tests in the following way:

- Start of the week: 100m sprint followed by (after a 5-10 min break or later in the day) 2km best effort – the strength tests can then be completed later in the day, but it would be ideal to perform them a day or two later.
- Complete the 3 strength tests on either separate days (as shown on the following program cards) or as a single session meet: 5RM Back Squat, Bench Press and Deadlift performed in 1 session (in that order).
- Complete the 10km best effort at the end of the week, ideally at least a couple of days after the strength tests.

If this week is not being used to test and is being used as a deload or taper week, follow the program cards (page-62-66) with the taper rep range on the primary lift.

Tribrid Program Card 16

Phase 3: 6-Week Testing – Week-1 (Week-6 of the program)

Conditioning Tests: I recommend completing the 100m Sprint and 2km Run/Row at the start of the week.

If you are not testing (deload or taper), I suggest going on a 1 hour walk or 15-20 min jog (RPE 3).

Strength Session 1: Primary Press

Exercise	Sets/Reps	Intensity	Rest	Notes
Optional: MB CM Chest Throw	3x1	Max Intent	5-10 Secs	Or Overhead (OH) CM Throw if doing a Strict/Push Press / Use a 3-5kg MB
BB Bench Press	5RM	Max	N/A	**Taper Sets & Reps:** 3x6 at RPE 5-6
Superset: Incline DB Press + DB Bent-Over Row	3x6+6	RPE 5-6	1-2 Mins	Take 5-10 seconds rest between the two exercises – 1-2 deep breaths
Superset: EZ Biceps Curl + EZ Skull Crusher	3x6+6	RPE 5-6	1-2 Mins	Take 5-10 seconds rest between the two exercises – 1-2 deep breaths
		RPE 6-7	10-30 Secs	Optional Core: Your choice from page-24

5RM Protocol:

You want to hit your 5RM within 5-6 sets – go for a 5RM with minimal breakdown in form (Training Max) – add 15% to this number (times the weight lifted by 1.15) and that is your 1RME (1 rep max estimate).

At this point, you should have a rough idea of what you might be able to lift for 5 reps, so here's an example of the progression towards a bench 5RM of 100kg:

1x10 at 20kg (unloaded barbell) – 1x6 at 40kg – 1x5 at 60kg – 1x3 at 85kg – First 5RM attempt at 100kg – rest for 3-5 minutes and if going for a 2nd attempt, add or take off the appropriate weight.

Note: I drop the reps below 5 on the final warm-up sets to stimulate the neuromuscular system without excessive fatigue.

Program Log 16:   Date: ____ / ____ / ____   Day: _____   Time: _____

Exercise	Set 1		Set 2		Set 3		Set 4		Set 5	
	WEIGHT		**WEIGHT**		**WEIGHT**		**WEIGHT**		**WEIGHT**	
	REP	RPE	REP	RPE	REP	RPE	REP	RPE	REP	RPE

Conditioning / Notes	Readiness	Bad	Ok	Good
	Sleep:			
	Energy:			
	Mood:			
	Soreness:			

Session RPE: _____

Tribrid Program Card 17

Phase 3: 6-Week Testing – Week-1 (Week-6 of the program)

Conditioning Tests: If you are not performing any of the tests (deload or taper), I suggest going on a 1 hour walk or 15-20 min jog (RPE 3).

Strength Session 2: Primary Deadlift

Exercise	Sets/Reps	Intensity	Rest	Notes
Optional: HCMJ	3x1	Max Intent	10-15 Secs	Horizontal (Broad) Countermovement Jump
BB Conventional Deadlift	5RM	Max	N/A	**Taper Sets & Reps:** 3x6 at RPE 5-6
Flat DB Press	3x6	RPE 5-6	1-2 Mins	Work at a steady tempo
Single-Arm Row	3x6 ES	RPE 5-6	1-2 Mins	Work at a steady tempo
		RPE 6-7	10-30 Secs	Optional Core: Your choice from page-24

5RM Protocol:

You want to hit your 5RM within 5-6 sets – go for a 5RM with minimal breakdown in form (Training Max) – add 15% to this number (times the weight lifted by 1.15) and that is your 1RME (1 rep max estimate).

At this point, you should have a rough idea of what you might be able to lift for 5 reps, so here's an example of the progression towards a deadlift 5RM of 160kg:

1x10 at 40kg (unloaded barbell) – 1x6 at 80kg – 1x5 at 100kg – 1x3 at 120kg – 1x2 at 140kg – First 5RM attempt at 160kg – rest for 3-5 minutes and if going for a 2nd attempt, add or take off the appropriate weight.

Note: I drop the reps below 5 on the final warm-up sets to stimulate the neuromuscular system without excessive fatigue.

Program Log 17:   Date: ____ / ____ / ____   Day: _____   Time: _____

Exercise	Set 1		Set 2		Set 3		Set 4		Set 5	
	WEIGHT		WEIGHT		WEIGHT		WEIGHT		WEIGHT	
	REP	RPE	REP	RPE	REP	RPE	REP	RPE	REP	RPE

Conditioning / Notes	Readiness	Bad	Ok	Good
	Sleep:			
	Energy:			
	Mood:			
	Soreness:			

Session RPE: _____

Tribrid Program Card 18

Phase 3: 6-Week Testing – Week-1 (Week-6 of the program)

Conditioning Tests: The 10km is best completed a couple of days after the final strength test.

If you are not performing any of the tests (deload or taper), I suggest going on a 1 hour walk or 15-20 min jog (RPE 3).

Strength Session 3: Primary Squat

Exercise	Sets/Reps	Intensity	Rest	Notes
Optional: VCMJ	3x1	Max Intent	10-15 Secs	Vertical Countermovement Jump
BB Back Squat	5RM	Max	N/A	**Taper Sets & Reps:** 3x6 at RPE 5-6
BB RDL	3x6	RPE 5-6	1-2 Mins	Work at a steady tempo
Seated DB Press	3x6	RPE 5-6	1-2 Mins	Work at a steady tempo
		RPE 6	10-30 Secs	Optional Core: Your choice from page-24

5RM Protocol:

You want to hit your 5RM within 5-6 sets – go for a 5RM with minimal breakdown in form (Training Max) – add 15% to this number (times the weight lifted by 1.15) and that is your 1RME (1 rep max estimate).

At this point, you should have a rough idea of what you might be able to lift for 5 reps, so here's an example of the progression towards a squat 5RM of 130kg:

1x10 at 20kg (unloaded barbell) – 1x6 at 50kg – 1x5 at 80kg – 1x3 at 100kg – 1x2 at 115kg – First 5RM attempt at 100kg – rest for 3-5 minutes and if going for a 2nd attempt, add or take off the appropriate weight.

Note: I drop the reps below 5 on the final warm-up sets to stimulate the neuromuscular system without excessive fatigue.

Program Log 18:   Date: ____ / ____ / ____   Day: _____   Time: _____

Exercise	Set 1 WEIGHT		Set 2 WEIGHT		Set 3 WEIGHT		Set 4 WEIGHT		Set 5 WEIGHT	
	REP	RPE	REP	RPE	REP	RPE	REP	RPE	REP	RPE

Conditioning / Notes	Readiness	Bad	Ok	Good
	Sleep:			
	Energy:			
	Mood:			
	Soreness:			

Session RPE: _____

Tribrid Program Card 19

Phase 4: Intensification – Week-1 (Week-7 of the program)

Strength Session 1: Primary Press

Clusters: When the reps are in brackets, it means 1 set includes several sets that are split by short breaks (place the barbell back on the J-cups): Ideal break for this week – 2 deep breaths in and out (around 10 seconds).

Exercise	Sets/Reps	Intensity	Rest	Notes
Optional: MB CM Chest Throw	5x1	Max Intent	5-10 Secs	Or Overhead (OH) CM Throw if doing a Strict/Push Press / Use a 3-5kg MB
BB Bench Press	3x(2x3)	RPE 9 (80%)	2-3 Mins	Lift fast and hard: Each set includes 2 sets of 3 reps with a 10 second break between them (2 deep breaths in and out)
Superset: Incline DB Press + DB Bent-Over Row	3x10+10	RPE 7-8	1-2 Mins	Work with a steady eccentric (steady down) and fast concentric (fast up)
Optional Superset: DB Fly + DB Bent-Over Lateral Raise	3x10+10	RPE 7-8	1-2 Mins	Work with a steady eccentric (steady down) and fast concentric (fast up)
Superset: EZ Biceps Curl + EZ Skull Crusher	3x10+10	RPE 7-8	1-2 Mins	Work with a steady eccentric (steady down) and fast concentric (fast up)
		RPE 7	10-30 Secs	Optional Core: Your choice from page-24

Conditioning Session 1: Speed (rest = between sets or the next distance).

Activity	Description	Rest
Run (Speed)	4x100m – 1st RPE 6 / 2nd RPE 8 / 3rd & 4th RPE 10	3 Mins
	3x200m – 1st RPE 9 / 2nd & 3rd RPE 8	2 Mins
	2x400m – RPE 7	2 Mins
Total Distance	1800m	N/A

Alternative: Perform distances on a rower or ski ERG or divide the distances by 10 and perform them as calories on an air bike (RPE 8) – follow the same rest periods (half them if on the air bike).

Program Log 19:   Date: ____ / ____ / ____   Day: _____   Time: _____

Exercise	Set 1 WEIGHT		Set 2 WEIGHT		Set 3 WEIGHT		Set 4 WEIGHT		Set 5 WEIGHT	
	REP	RPE	REP	RPE	REP	RPE	REP	RPE	REP	RPE

Conditioning / Notes	Readiness	Bad	Ok	Good
	Sleep:			
	Energy:			
	Mood:			
	Soreness:			

Session RPE: _____

Tribrid Program Card 20

Phase 4: Intensification – Week-1 (Week-7 of the program)

Strength Session 2: Primary Deadlift

Clusters: When the reps are in brackets, it means 1 set includes several sets that are split by short breaks (place the barbell on the floor): Ideal break for this week – 2 deep breaths in and out (around 10 seconds).

Exercise	Sets/Reps	Intensity	Rest	Notes
Optional: H Hop	3x1 ES	Max Intent	10-15 Secs	Horizontal Hops – jump forward from one leg and land on the same leg
BB Conventional Deadlift	3x(2x3)	RPE 9 (80%)	2-3 Mins	Lift fast and hard: Each set includes 2 sets of 3 reps with a 10 second break between them (2 deep breaths in and out)
DB RFESS	3x10 ES	RPE 7-8	1-2 Mins	Work with a steady eccentric (steady down) and fast concentric (fast up)
Flat DB Press	3x10	RPE 7-8	1-2 Mins	Work with a steady eccentric (steady down) and fast concentric (fast up)
Single-Arm Row	3x10 ES	RPE 7-8	1-2 Mins	Work with a steady eccentric (steady down) and fast concentric (fast up)
		RPE 7	10-30 Secs	Optional Core: Your choice from page-24

Conditioning Session 2: Tempo

Activity	Description
Run/Row (Tempo)	2x3km Run/Row – RPE 8-9 (Push the pace) 5 Mins rest between sets

Alternative: Perform 6x40 Secs Work, 20 Secs Rest (RPE 9) on a cardio machine (rower, bike, etc), or on equipment such as battle ropes, slam balls or the prowler, etc (post SS2 or another time).

Program Log 20: Date: ____ / ____ / ____ Day: _____ Time: _____

Exercise	Set 1		Set 2		Set 3		Set 4		Set 5	
	WEIGHT		WEIGHT		WEIGHT		WEIGHT		WEIGHT	
	REP	RPE	REP	RPE	REP	RPE	REP	RPE	REP	RPE

Conditioning / Notes	Readiness	Bad	Ok	Good
	Sleep:			
	Energy:			
	Mood:			
	Soreness:			

Session RPE: _____

Tribrid Program Card 21

Phase 4: Intensification – Week-1 (Week-7 of the program)

Strength Session 3: Primary Squat

Clusters: When the reps are in brackets, it means 1 set includes several sets that are split by short breaks (place the barbell back on the J-cups): Ideal break for this week – 2 deep breaths in and out (around 10 seconds).

Exercise	Sets/Reps	Intensity	Rest	Notes
Optional: Pogo Jump	3x10	Max Intent	10-15 Secs	Vertical jump with your hands on your hips – emphasis on ankles and knees
BB Back Squat	3x(2x3)	RPE 9 (80%)	2-3 Mins	Lift fast and hard: Each set includes 2 sets of 3 reps with a 10 second break between them (2 deep breaths in and out)
BB RDL	3x10	RPE 7-8	1-2 Mins	Work with a steady eccentric (steady down) and fast concentric (fast up)
Seated DB Press	3x10	RPE 7-8	1-2 Mins	Work with a steady eccentric (steady down) and fast concentric (fast up)
Pull-Up	3xMax	RPE 10	1-2 Mins	Resistance band(s) can be used to regress the movement or weight can be added to progress it – aim for a min of 2 reps and a max of 10 if using bands
		RPE 7	10-30 Secs	Optional Core: Your choice from page-24

Conditioning Session 3: Steady State

Activity	Description
Run/Row (Steady State)	6km Run/Row – RPE 4

Alternative: Perform 6x40 Secs Work, 20 Secs Rest (RPE 9) on a cardio machine (rower, bike, etc), or on equipment such as battle ropes, slam balls or the prowler, etc (post SS3 or another time).

Program Log 21:   Date: ____ / ____ / ____   Day: _____   Time: _____

Exercise	Set 1 WEIGHT		Set 2 WEIGHT		Set 3 WEIGHT		Set 4 WEIGHT		Set 5 WEIGHT	
	REP	RPE	REP	RPE	REP	RPE	REP	RPE	REP	RPE

Conditioning / Notes	Readiness	Bad	Ok	Good
	Sleep:			
	Energy:			
	Mood:			
	Soreness:			

Session RPE: _____

Tribrid Program Card 22

Phase 4: Intensification – Week-2 (Week-8 of the program)

Strength Session 1: Primary Press

Clusters: When the reps are in brackets, it means 1 set includes several sets that are split by short breaks (place the barbell back on the J-cups): Ideal break for this week – 2-3 deep breaths in and out (around 10-15 seconds).

Exercise	Sets/Reps	Intensity	Rest	Notes
Optional: MB CM Chest Throw	5x1	Max Intent	5-10 Secs	Or Overhead (OH) CM Throw if doing a Strict/Push Press / Use a 3-5kg MB
BB Bench Press	3x(3x2)	RPE 9-10 (85%)	2-3 Mins	Lift fast and hard: Each set includes 3 sets of 2 reps with a 10-15 second break between them (2-3 deep breaths in and out)
Superset: Incline DB Press + DB Bent-Over Row	3x8+8	RPE 8-9	1-2 Mins	Work with a steady eccentric (steady down) and fast concentric (fast up)
Optional Superset: DB Fly + DB Bent-Over Lateral Raise	3x8+8	RPE 8-9	1-2 Mins	Work with a steady eccentric (steady down) and fast concentric (fast up)
Superset: EZ Biceps Curl + EZ Skull Crusher	3x8+8	RPE 8-9	1-2 Mins	Work with a steady eccentric (steady down) and fast concentric (fast up)
		RPE 7	10-30 Secs	Optional Core: Your choice from page-24

Conditioning Session 1: Speed (rest = between sets or the next distance).

Activity	Description	Rest
Run (Speed)	4x100m – 1st RPE 6 / 2nd RPE 8 / 3rd & 4th RPE 10	3 Mins
	3x200m – 1st RPE 9 / 2nd & 3rd RPE 8	3 Mins
	1x400m – RPE 10	N/A
Total Distance	1400m	N/A

Alternative: Perform distances on a rower or ski ERG or divide the distances by 10 and perform them as calories on an air bike (RPE 8) – follow the same rest periods (half them if on the air bike).

Program Log 22: Date: ____ / ____ / ____ Day: _____ Time: _____

Exercise	Set 1 WEIGHT		Set 2 WEIGHT		Set 3 WEIGHT		Set 4 WEIGHT		Set 5 WEIGHT	
	REP	RPE	REP	RPE	REP	RPE	REP	RPE	REP	RPE

Conditioning / Notes	Readiness	Bad	Ok	Good
	Sleep:			
	Energy:			
	Mood:			
	Soreness:			

Session RPE: _____

Tribrid Program Card 23

Phase 4: Intensification – Week-2 (Week-8 of the program)

Strength Session 2: Primary Deadlift

Clusters: When the reps are in brackets, it means 1 set includes several sets that are split by short breaks (place the barbell on the floor): Ideal break for this week – 2-3 deep breaths in and out (around 10-15 seconds).

Exercise	Sets/Reps	Intensity	Rest	Notes
Optional: H Hop	3x2 ES	Max Intent	10-15 Secs	Horizontal Hops – jump forward from one leg and land on the same leg
BB Conventional Deadlift	3x(3x2)	RPE 9-10 (85%)	2-3 Mins	Lift fast and hard: Each set includes 3 sets of 2 reps with a 10-15 second break between them (2-3 deep breaths in and out)
DB RFESS	3x8 ES	RPE 8-9	1-2 Mins	Work with a steady eccentric (steady down) and fast concentric (fast up)
Flat DB Press	3x8	RPE 8-9	1-2 Mins	Work with a steady eccentric (steady down) and fast concentric (fast up)
Single-Arm Row	3x8 ES	RPE 8-9	1-2 Mins	Work with a steady eccentric (steady down) and fast concentric (fast up)
		RPE 7	10-30 Secs	Optional Core: Your choice from page-24

Conditioning Session 2: Tempo

Activity	Description
Run/Row (Tempo)	3x2km Run/Row – RPE 9 (Push the pace) 5 Mins rest between sets

Alternative: Perform 8x30 Secs Work, 15 Secs Rest (RPE 10) on a cardio machine (rower, bike, etc), or on equipment such as battle ropes, slam balls or the prowler, etc (post SS2 or another time).

Program Log 23:   Date: ____ / ____ / ____   Day: _____   Time: _____

Exercise	Set 1		Set 2		Set 3		Set 4		Set 5	
	WEIGHT		WEIGHT		WEIGHT		WEIGHT		WEIGHT	
	REP	RPE	REP	RPE	REP	RPE	REP	RPE	REP	RPE

Conditioning / Notes	Readiness	Bad	Ok	Good
	Sleep:			
	Energy:			
	Mood:			
	Soreness:			

Session RPE: _____

Tribrid Program Card 24

Phase 4: Intensification – Week-2 (Week-8 of the program)

Strength Session 3: Primary Squat

Clusters: When the reps are in brackets, it means 1 set includes several sets that are split by short breaks (place the barbell back on the J-cups): Ideal break for this week – 2-3 deep breaths in and out (around 10-15 seconds).

Exercise	Sets/Reps	Intensity	Rest	Notes
Optional: Pogo Jump	3x10	Max Intent	10-15 Secs	Vertical jump with your hands on your hips – emphasis on ankles and knees
BB Back Squat	3x(3x2)	RPE 9-10 (85%)	2-3 Mins	Lift fast and hard: Each set includes 3 sets of 2 reps with a 10-15 second break between them (2-3 deep breaths in and out)
BB RDL	3x8	RPE 8-9	1-2 Mins	Work with a steady eccentric (steady down) and fast concentric (fast up)
Seated DB Press	3x8	RPE 8-9	1-2 Mins	Work with a steady eccentric (steady down) and fast concentric (fast up)
Pull-Up	3xMax	RPE 10	1-2 Mins	Resistance band(s) can be used to regress the movement or weight can be added to progress it – aim for a min of 2 reps and a max of 10 if using bands
		RPE 7	10-30 Secs	Optional Core: Your choice from page-24

Conditioning Session 3: Steady State

Activity	Description
Run/Row (Steady State)	10km Run/Row – RPE 4-5

Alternative: Perform 8x30 Secs Work, 15 Secs Rest (RPE 10) on a cardio machine (rower, bike, etc), or on equipment such as battle ropes, slam balls or the prowler, etc (post SS3 or another time).

Program Log 24:   Date: ____ / ____ / ____   Day: _____   Time: _____

Exercise	Set 1 WEIGHT		Set 2 WEIGHT		Set 3 WEIGHT		Set 4 WEIGHT		Set 5 WEIGHT	
	REP	RPE	REP	RPE	REP	RPE	REP	RPE	REP	RPE

Conditioning / Notes	Readiness	Bad	Ok	Good
	Sleep:			
	Energy:			
	Mood:			
	Soreness:			

Session RPE: _____

Tribrid Program Card 25

Phase 4: Intensification – Week-3 (Week-9 of the program)

Strength Session 1: Primary Press

Clusters: When the reps are in brackets, it means 1 set includes several sets that are split by short breaks (place the barbell back on the J-cups): Ideal break for this week – 3 deep breaths in and out (around 15 seconds).

Exercise	Sets/Reps	Intensity	Rest	Notes
Optional: MB CM Chest Throw	5x1	Max Intent	5-10 Secs	Or Overhead (OH) CM Throw if doing a Strict/Push Press / Use a 3-5kg MB
BB Bench Press	3x(2x2)	RPE 10 (90%)	2-3 Mins	Lift fast and hard: Each set includes 2 sets of 2 reps with a 15 second break between them (3 deep breaths in and out)
Superset: Incline DB Press + DB Bent-Over Row	3x6+6	RPE 9	1-2 Mins	Work with a steady eccentric (steady down) and fast concentric (fast up)
Optional Superset: DB Fly + DB Bent-Over Lateral Raise	3x6+6	RPE 9	1-2 Mins	Work with a steady eccentric (steady down) and fast concentric (fast up)
Superset: EZ Biceps Curl + EZ Skull Crusher	3x6+6	RPE 9	1-2 Mins	Work with a steady eccentric (steady down) and fast concentric (fast up)
		RPE 7	10-30 Secs	Optional Core: Your choice from page-24

Conditioning Session 1: Speed (rest = between sets or the next distance).

Activity	Description	Rest
Run (Speed)	4x100m – 1st RPE 7 / 2nd RPE 9 / 3rd & 4th RPE 10	3 Mins
	3x200m – RPE 10	3 Mins
Total Distance	1000m	N/A

Alternative: Perform distances on a rower or ski ERG or divide the distances by 10 and perform them as calories on an air bike (RPE 8) – follow the same rest periods (half them if on the air bike).

Program Log 25:   Date: ____ / ____ / ____   Day: _____   Time: _____

Exercise	Set 1		Set 2		Set 3		Set 4		Set 5	
	WEIGHT		WEIGHT		WEIGHT		WEIGHT		WEIGHT	
	REP	RPE	REP	RPE	REP	RPE	REP	RPE	REP	RPE

Conditioning / Notes	Readiness	Bad	Ok	Good
	Sleep:			
	Energy:			
	Mood:			
	Soreness:			

Session RPE: _____

Tribrid Program Card 26

Phase 4: Intensification – Week-3 (Week-9 of the program)

Strength Session 2: Primary Deadlift

Clusters: When the reps are in brackets, it means 1 set includes several sets that are split by short breaks (place the barbell on the floor): Ideal break for this week – 3 deep breaths in and out (around 15 seconds).

Exercise	Sets/Reps	Intensity	Rest	Notes
Optional: Horizontal CM Hop	3x3 ES	Max Intent	10-15 Secs	Horizontal Hops – jump forward from one leg and land on the same leg
BB Conventional Deadlift	3x(2x2)	RPE 10 (90%)	2-3 Mins	Lift fast and hard: Each set includes 2 sets of 2 reps with a 10-15 second break between them (2-3 deep breaths in and out)
DB RFESS	3x6 ES	RPE 9	1-2 Mins	Work with a steady eccentric (steady down) and fast concentric (fast up)
Flat DB Press	3x6	RPE 9	1-2 Mins	Work with a steady eccentric (steady down) and fast concentric (fast up)
Single-Arm Row	3x6 ES	RPE 9	1-2 Mins	Work with a steady eccentric (steady down) and fast concentric (fast up)
		RPE 7	10-30 Secs	Optional Core: Your choice from page-24

Conditioning Session 2: Tempo

Activity	Description
Run/Row (Tempo)	2x1km Run/Row – RPE 10 5 Mins rest between sets

Alternative: Perform 10x20 Secs Work, 10 Secs Rest (RPE 10) on a cardio machine (rower, bike, etc), or on equipment such as battle ropes, slam balls or the prowler, etc (post SS2 or another time).

Program Log 26:   Date: ____ / ____ / ____   Day: _____   Time: _____

Exercise	Set 1 WEIGHT		Set 2 WEIGHT		Set 3 WEIGHT		Set 4 WEIGHT		Set 5 WEIGHT	
	REP	RPE	REP	RPE	REP	RPE	REP	RPE	REP	RPE

Conditioning / Notes	Readiness	Bad	Ok	Good
	Sleep:			
	Energy:			
	Mood:			
	Soreness:			

Session RPE: _____

Tribrid Program Card 27

Phase 4: Intensification – Week-2 (Week-8 of the program)

Strength Session 3: Primary Squat

Clusters: When the reps are in brackets, it means 1 set includes several sets that are split by short breaks (place the barbell back on the J-cups): Ideal break for this week – 2-3 deep breaths in and out (around 10-15 seconds).

Exercise	Sets/Reps	Intensity	Rest	Notes
Optional: Pogo Jump	3x10	Max Intent	10-15 Secs	Vertical jump with your hands on your hips – emphasis on ankles and knees
BB Back Squat	3x(2x2)	RPE 10 (90%)	2-3 Mins	Lift fast and hard: Each set includes 2 sets of 2 reps with a 10-15 second break between them (2-3 deep breaths in and out)
BB RDL	3x6	RPE 9	1-2 Mins	Work with a steady eccentric (steady down) and fast concentric (fast up)
Seated DB Press	3x6	RPE 9	1-2 Mins	Work with a steady eccentric (steady down) and fast concentric (fast up)
Pull-Up	3xMax	RPE 10	1-2 Mins	Resistance band(s) can be used to regress the movement or weight can be added to progress it – aim for a min of 2 reps and a max of 10 if using bands
		RPE 7	10-30 Secs	Optional Core: Your choice from page-24

Conditioning Session 3: Steady State

Activity	Description
Run/Row (Steady State)	12km Run/Row – RPE 5-6

Alternative: Perform 10x20 Secs Work, 10 Secs Rest (RPE 10) on a cardio machine (rower, bike, etc), or on equipment such as battle ropes, slam balls or the prowler, etc (post SS3 or another time).

Program Log 27: Date: ____ / ____ / ____ Day: _____ Time: _____

Exercise	Set 1 WEIGHT		Set 2 WEIGHT		Set 3 WEIGHT		Set 4 WEIGHT		Set 5 WEIGHT	
	REP	RPE	REP	RPE	REP	RPE	REP	RPE	REP	RPE

Conditioning / Notes	Readiness	Bad	Ok	Good
	Sleep:			
	Energy:			
	Mood:			
	Soreness:			

Session RPE: _____

Tribrid Program Card 28

Phase 5: Realization – Week-1 (Week-10 of the program)

Strength Session 1: Primary Press

Complex Training: A heavy strength lift is followed by a ballistic/plyometric exercise – Bench Press into MB Countermovement Chest Throw (10-15 second break between them – 2-3 deep breaths in and out).

Exercise	Sets/Reps	Intensity	Rest	Notes
Optional: MB Single-Arm CM Chest Throw	3x1	Max Intent	5-10 Secs	Or Overhead (OH) CM Throw if doing a Strict/Push Press / Use a 3-5kg MB
BB Bench Press + MB CM Chest Throw	3x3+3	RPE 10 (85%)	2-3 Mins	Lift fast and hard: Perform 3 heavy presses followed by 3 countermovement chest throws with a 3-5kg MB
Superset: Incline DB Press + DB Bent-Over Row	3x5+5	RPE 9	1-2 Mins	Lift fast and hard
Optional Superset: DB Fly + DB Bent-Over Lateral Raise	3x5+5	RPE 9	1-2 Mins	Lift fast and hard
Superset: EZ Biceps Curl + EZ Skull Crusher	3x5+5	RPE 9	1-2 Mins	Lift fast and hard
		RPE 7	10-30 Secs	Optional Core: Your choice from page-24

Conditioning Session 1: Speed (rest = between sets or the next distance).

Activity	Description	Rest
Run (Speed)	4x100m – 1st RPE 7 / 3rd, 4th & 5th RPE 10	3 Mins
	2x200m – RPE 10	3 Mins
Total Distance	800m	N/A

Alternative: Perform distances on a rower or ski ERG or divide the distances by 10 and perform them as calories on an air bike (RPE 8) – follow the same rest periods (half them if on the air bike).

Program Log 28:   Date: ____ / ____ / ____   Day: _____   Time: _____

Exercise	Set 1 WEIGHT		Set 2 WEIGHT		Set 3 WEIGHT		Set 4 WEIGHT		Set 5 WEIGHT	
	REP	RPE	REP	RPE	REP	RPE	REP	RPE	REP	RPE

Conditioning / Notes	Readiness	Bad	Ok	Good
	Sleep:			
	Energy:			
	Mood:			
	Soreness:			

Session RPE: _____

Tribrid Program Card 29

Phase 5: Realization – Week-1 (Week-10 of the program)

Strength Session 2: Primary Deadlift

Complex Training: A heavy strength lift is followed by a ballistic/plyometric exercise – Deadlift into Horizontal Countermovement Jump (10-15 second break between them – 2-3 deep breaths in and out).

Exercise	Sets/Reps	Intensity	Rest	Notes
Optional: Bounds	3x3 ES	Max Intent	10-15 Secs	Horizontal Hops – jump forward from one leg and land on the same leg
BB Conventional Deadlift + Horizontal CM Jump	3x3+3	RPE 10 (85%)	2-3 Mins	Lift fast and hard: Perform 3 heavy deadlifts followed by 3 horizontal jumps
DB RFESS	3x5 ES	RPE 9	1-2 Mins	Lift fast and hard
Flat DB Press	3x5	RPE 9	1-2 Mins	Lift fast and hard
Single-Arm Row	3x5 ES	RPE 9	1-2 Mins	Lift fast and hard
		RPE 7	10-30 Secs	Optional Core: Your choice from page-24

Conditioning Session 2: Tempo

Activity	Description
Run/Row (Tempo)	2x1km Run/Row – RPE 10 5 Mins rest between sets

Alternative: Perform 8x20 Secs Work, 20 Secs Rest (RPE 10) on a cardio machine (rower, bike, etc), or on equipment such as battle ropes, slam balls or the prowler, etc (post SS2 or another time).

Program Log 29:   Date: ___ / ___ / ___   Day: _____   Time: _____

Exercise	Set 1 WEIGHT		Set 2 WEIGHT		Set 3 WEIGHT		Set 4 WEIGHT		Set 5 WEIGHT	
	REP	RPE	REP	RPE	REP	RPE	REP	RPE	REP	RPE

Conditioning / Notes	Readiness	Bad	Ok	Good
	Sleep:			
	Energy:			
	Mood:			
	Soreness:			

Session RPE: _____

Tribrid Program Card 30

Phase 5: Realization – Week-1 (Week-10 of the program)

Strength Session 3: Primary Squat

Complex Training: A heavy strength lift is followed by a ballistic/plyometric exercise – Squat into Vertical Countermovement Jump (10-15 second break between them – 2-3 deep breaths in and out).

Exercise	Sets/Reps	Intensity	Rest	Notes
Optional: Ankle Jump	3x10	Max Intent	10-15 Secs	Vertical jump with your hands on your hips – emphasis on ankles
BB Back Squat	3x3+3	RPE 10 (85%)	2-3 Mins	Lift fast and hard: Perform 3 heavy squats followed by 3 vertical jumps
BB RDL	3x5	RPE 9	1-2 Mins	Lift fast and hard
Seated DB Press	3x5	RPE 9	1-2 Mins	Lift fast and hard
Pull-Up	3xMax	RPE 10	1-2 Mins	Resistance band(s) can be used to regress the movement or weight can be added to progress it – aim for a min of 2 reps and a max of 10 if using bands
		RPE 7	10-30 Secs	Optional Core: Your choice from page-24

Conditioning Session 3: Steady State

Activity	Description
Run/Row (Steady State)	8km Run/Row – RPE 4-5

Alternative: Perform 8x20 Secs Work, 20 Secs Rest (RPE 10) on a cardio machine (rower, bike, etc), or on equipment such as battle ropes, slam balls or the prowler, etc (post SS3 or another time).

Program Log 30:   Date: ____ / ____ / ____   Day: _____ Time: _____

Exercise	Set 1 WEIGHT		Set 2 WEIGHT		Set 3 WEIGHT		Set 4 WEIGHT		Set 5 WEIGHT	
	REP	RPE	REP	RPE	REP	RPE	REP	RPE	REP	RPE

Conditioning / Notes	Readiness	Bad	Ok	Good
	Sleep:			
	Energy:			
	Mood:			
	Soreness:			

Session RPE: _____

Tribrid Program Card 31

Phase 5: Realization – Week-2 (Week-11 of the program)

Strength Session 1: Primary Press

Complex Training: A heavy strength lift is followed by a ballistic/plyometric exercise – Bench Press into MB Countermovement Chest Throw (10-15 second break between them – 2-3 deep breaths in and out).

Exercise	Sets/Reps	Intensity	Rest	Notes
Optional: MB Single-Arm CM Chest Throw	3x1	Max Intent	5-10 Secs	Or Overhead (OH) CM Throw if doing a Strict/Push Press / Use a 3-5kg MB
BB Bench Press + MB CM Chest Throw	3x2+2	RPE 10 (90%)	2-3 Mins	Lift fast and hard: Perform 2 heavy presses followed by 2 countermovement chest throws with a 3-5kg MB
Superset: Incline DB Press + DB Bent-Over Row	3x4+4	RPE 9-10	1-2 Mins	Lift fast and hard
Optional Superset: DB Fly + DB Bent-Over Lateral Raise	3x4+4	RPE 9-10	1-2 Mins	Lift fast and hard
Superset: EZ Biceps Curl + EZ Skull Crusher	3x4+4	RPE 9-10	1-2 Mins	Lift fast and hard
		RPE 7	10-30 Secs	Optional Core: Your choice from page-24

Conditioning Session 1: Speed (rest = between sets or the next distance).

Activity	Description	Rest
Run (Speed)	4x100m – 1st RPE 7 / 3rd, 4th & 5th RPE 10	3 Mins
Total Distance	400m	N/A

Alternative: Perform distances on a rower or ski ERG or divide the distances by 10 and perform them as calories on an air bike (RPE 8) – follow the same rest periods (half them if on the air bike).

Program Log 31: Date: ____ / ____ / ____ Day: _____ Time: _____

Exercise	Set 1		Set 2		Set 3		Set 4		Set 5	
	WEIGHT		*WEIGHT*		*WEIGHT*		*WEIGHT*		*WEIGHT*	
	REP	*RPE*	*REP*	*RPE*	*REP*	*RPE*	*REP*	*RPE*	*REP*	*RPE*

Conditioning / Notes	Readiness	Bad	Ok	Good
	Sleep:			
	Energy:			
	Mood:			
	Soreness:			

Session RPE: _____

Tribrid Program Card 32

Phase 5: Realization – Week-2 (Week-11 of the program)

Strength Session 2: Primary Deadlift

Complex Training: A heavy strength lift is followed by a ballistic/plyometric exercise – Deadlift into Horizontal Countermovement Jump (10-15 second break between them – 2-3 deep breaths in and out).

Exercise	Sets/Reps	Intensity	Rest	Notes
Optional: Bounds	3x3 ES	Max Intent	10-15 Secs	Horizontal Hops – jump forward from one leg and land on the same leg
BB Conventional Deadlift + Horizontal CM Jump	3x2+2	RPE 10 (90%)	2-3 Mins	Lift fast and hard: Perform 2 heavy deadlifts followed by 2 horizontal jumps
DB RFESS	3x4 ES	RPE 9-10	1-2 Mins	Lift fast and hard
Flat DB Press	3x4	RPE 9-10	1-2 Mins	Lift fast and hard
Single-Arm Row	3x4 ES	RPE 9-10	1-2 Mins	Lift fast and hard
		RPE 7	10-30 Secs	Optional Core: Your choice from page-24

Conditioning Session 2: Tempo

Activity	Description
Run/Row (Tempo)	1km Run/Row – RPE 10

Alternative: Perform 8x20 Secs Work, 30 Secs Rest (RPE 10) on a cardio machine (rower, bike, etc), or on equipment such as battle ropes, slam balls or the prowler, etc (post SS2 or another time).

Program Log 32:   Date: ____ / ____ / ____   Day: _____   Time: _____

Exercise	Set 1 WEIGHT		Set 2 WEIGHT		Set 3 WEIGHT		Set 4 WEIGHT		Set 5 WEIGHT	
	REP	RPE	REP	RPE	REP	RPE	REP	RPE	REP	RPE

Conditioning / Notes	Readiness	Bad	Ok	Good
	Sleep:			
	Energy:			
	Mood:			
	Soreness:			

Session RPE: _____

Tribrid Program Card 33

Phase 5: Realization – Week-2 (Week-11 of the program)

Strength Session 3: Primary Squat

Complex Training: A heavy strength lift is followed by a ballistic/plyometric exercise – Squat into Vertical Countermovement Jump (10-15 second break between them – 2-3 deep breaths in and out).

Exercise	Sets/Reps	Intensity	Rest	Notes
Optional: Ankle Jump	3x10	Max Intent	10-15 Secs	Vertical jump with your hands on your hips – emphasis on ankles
BB Back Squat	3x2+2	RPE 10 (90%)	2-3 Mins	Lift fast and hard: Perform 2 heavy squats followed by 2 vertical jumps
BB RDL	3x4	RPE 9-10	1-2 Mins	Lift fast and hard
Seated DB Press	3x4	RPE 9-10	1-2 Mins	Lift fast and hard
Pull-Up	3xMax	RPE 10	1-2 Mins	Resistance band(s) can be used to regress the movement or weight can be added to progress it – aim for a min of 2 reps and a max of 10 if using bands
		RPE 7	10-30 Secs	Optional Core: Your choice from page-24

Conditioning Session 3: Steady State

Activity	Description
Run/Row (Steady State)	5km Run/Row – RPE 4-5

Alternative: Perform 8x20 Secs Work, 30 Secs Rest (RPE 10) on a cardio machine (rower, bike, etc), or on equipment such as battle ropes, slam balls or the prowler, etc (post SS3 or another time).

Program Log 33:   Date: ____ / ____ / ____   Day: _____   Time: _____

Exercise	Set 1 WEIGHT		Set 2 WEIGHT		Set 3 WEIGHT		Set 4 WEIGHT		Set 5 WEIGHT	
	REP	RPE	REP	RPE	REP	RPE	REP	RPE	REP	RPE

Conditioning / Notes	Readiness	Bad	Ok	Good
	Sleep:			
	Energy:			
	Mood:			
	Soreness:			

Session RPE: _____

Week-12 Testing/Taper

During week-12 testing, there are 6 tests to complete.

1. 1RM Back Squat
2. 1RM Bench Press
3. 1RM Deadlift
4. 100m Sprint
5. 2km Run or Row
6. 10km Run or Row

I suggest completing the tests in the following way:

- Start of the week: 100m sprint followed by (after a 5-10 min break or later in the day) 2km best effort – the strength tests can then be completed later in the day, but it would be ideal to perform them a day or two later.
- Complete the 3 strength tests on either separate days (as shown on the following program cards) or as a single session meet: 1RM Back Squat, Bench Press and Deadlift performed in 1 session (in that order).
- Complete the 10km best effort at the end of the week, ideally at least a couple of days after the strength tests.

If this week is not being used to test and is being used as a deload or taper week, follow the program cards (page-100-104) with the taper rep range on the primary lift.

Tribrid Program Card 34

Phase 6: 12-Week Testing – Week-1 (Week-12 of the program)

Conditioning Tests: I recommend completing the 100m Sprint and 2km Run/Row at the start of the week.

If you are not testing (deload or taper), I suggest going on a 1 hour walk or 15-20 min jog (RPE 3).

Strength Session 1: Primary Press

Exercise	Sets/Reps	Intensity	Rest	Notes
Optional: MB CM Chest Throw	3x1	Max Intent	5-10 Secs	Or Overhead (OH) CM Throw if doing a Strict/Push Press / Use a 3-5kg MB
BB Bench Press	1RM	Max	N/A	**Taper Sets & Reps:** 3x6 at RPE 5-6
Superset: Incline DB Press + DB Bent-Over Row	3x6+6	RPE 5-6	1-2 Mins	Take 5-10 seconds rest between the two exercises – 1-2 deep breaths
Superset: EZ Biceps Curl + EZ Skull Crusher	3x6+6	RPE 5-6	1-2 Mins	Take 5-10 seconds rest between the two exercises – 1-2 deep breaths
		RPE 6-7	10-30 Secs	Optional Core: Your choice from page-24

1RM Protocol:

You want to hit your 1RM within 5-6 sets.

At this point, you should have a rough idea of what your 1RM might be, so here's an example of the progression towards a bench 1RM of 120kg:

1x10 at 20kg (unloaded barbell) – 1x6 at 50kg – 1x3 at 70kg – 1x1 at 100kg – 1x1 at 110kg – First 1RM attempt at 120kg – rest for 3-5 minutes and if going for a 2nd attempt, add or take off the appropriate weight.

Date: ____ / ____ / ____ Day: _____ Time: _____

Exercise	Set 1 WEIGHT		Set 2 WEIGHT		Set 3 WEIGHT		Set 4 WEIGHT		Set 5 WEIGHT	
	REP	RPE	REP	RPE	REP	RPE	REP	RPE	REP	RPE

Conditioning / Notes	Readiness	Bad	Ok	Good
	Sleep:			
	Energy:			
	Mood:			
	Soreness:			

Session RPE: _____

Tribrid Program Card 35

Phase 6: 12-Week Testing – Week-1 (Week-12 of the program)

Conditioning Tests: If you are not performing any of the tests (deload or taper), I suggest going on a 1 hour walk or 15-20 min jog (RPE 3).

Strength Session 2: Primary Deadlift

Exercise	Sets/Reps	Intensity	Rest	Notes
Optional: HCMJ	3x1	Max Intent	10-15 Secs	Horizontal (Broad) Countermovement Jump
BB Conventional Deadlift	1RM	Max	N/A	**Taper Sets & Reps:** 3x6 at RPE 5-6
Flat DB Press	3x6	RPE 5-6	1-2 Mins	Work at a steady tempo
Single-Arm Row	3x6 ES	RPE 5-6	1-2 Mins	Work at a steady tempo
		RPE 6-7	10-30 Secs	Optional Core: Your choice from page-24

1RM Protocol:

You want to hit your 1RM within 5-6 sets.

At this point, you should have a rough idea of what your 1RM might be, so here's an example of the progression toward a deadlift 1RM of 200kg:

1x8 at 60kg (unloaded barbell) – 1x5 at 100kg – 1x3 at 140kg – 1x2 at 160kg – 1x1 at 180kg – First 1RM attempt at 200kg – rest for 3-5 minutes and if going for a 2nd attempt, add or take off the appropriate weight.

Program Log 35:   Date: ____ / ____ / ____   Day: _____   Time: _____

Exercise	Set 1 WEIGHT		Set 2 WEIGHT		Set 3 WEIGHT		Set 4 WEIGHT		Set 5 WEIGHT	
	REP	RPE	REP	RPE	REP	RPE	REP	RPE	REP	RPE

Conditioning / Notes	Readiness	Bad	Ok	Good
	Sleep:			
	Energy:			
	Mood:			
	Soreness:			

Session RPE: _____

Tribrid Program Card 36

Phase 6: 12-Week Testing – Week-1 (Week-12 of the program)

Conditioning Tests: The 10km is best completed a couple of days after the final strength test.

If you are not performing any of the tests (deload or taper), I suggest going on a 1 hour walk or 15-20 min jog (RPE 3).

Strength Session 3: Primary Squat

Exercise	Sets/Reps	Intensity	Rest	Notes
Optional: VCMJ	3x1	Max Intent	10-15 Secs	Vertical Countermovement Jump
BB Back Squat	1RM	Max	N/A	**Taper Sets & Reps:** 3x6 at RPE 5-6
BB RDL	3x6	RPE 5-6	1-2 Mins	Work at a steady tempo
Seated DB Press	3x6	RPE 5-6	1-2 Mins	Work at a steady tempo
		RPE 6	10-30 Secs	Optional Core: Your choice from page-24

1RM Protocol:

You want to hit your 1RM within 5-6 sets.

At this point, you should have a rough idea of what your 1RM might be, so here's an example of the progression towards a squat 1RM of 160kg:

1x10 at 20kg (unloaded barbell) – 1x8 at 60kg – 1x5 at 100kg – 1x2 at 120kg – 1x1 at 140kg – First 1RM attempt at 160kg – rest for 3-5 minutes and if going for a 2nd attempt, add or take off the appropriate weight.

Program Log 36:   Date: ____ / ____ / ____ Day: _____ Time: _____

Exercise	Set 1 WEIGHT		Set 2 WEIGHT		Set 3 WEIGHT		Set 4 WEIGHT		Set 5 WEIGHT	
	REP	RPE	REP	RPE	REP	RPE	REP	RPE	REP	RPE

Conditioning / Notes	Readiness	Bad	Ok	Good
	Sleep:			
	Energy:			
	Mood:			
	Soreness:			

Session RPE: _____

Final Thoughts

Firstly, thanks for downloading a copy of my flagship program: Tribrid Training.

Over many years of owning a strength and conditioning gym, working with athletes of all levels, the military, and literally 1000's of clients from the general population, I have identified numerous key elements to good programming.

Individualization is an important training principle. However, 99.9% of people simply need the fundamentals of each training mode executed in a structured and well-thought-out way.

The aim of Tribrid Training is to provide that structure for the 3-Key-Qualities: Strength – Speed – Stamina. A program that ticks all the right boxes and has a clear progression, but also allows for flexibility in terms of the training split and exercise selection.

I would love to hear your thoughts on the Tribrid System (both things you found positive and negative), so please drop me an email at jay@scc.coach and I will answer all emails personally.

Following this page, I have included examples of some of my most popular content – the QR code on the final pages directs you to my LinkTree with over 600-pages of FREE content (you can also check out my books and online courses).

Thanks Again,

Coach Curtis

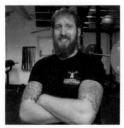

Helpful FREE Content!

Link and QR Code on the last page.

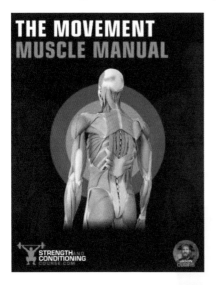

This unique muscle manual categorizes muscles by their movements, giving you a much better understanding of how muscles assist and oppose each other to perform movements.

You also get a FREE second version of the muscle manual, which lists muscle origins, insertions, nerve innervations, etc.

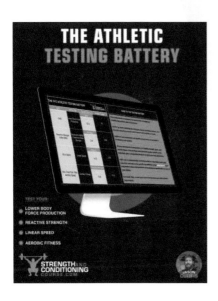

This excel tool tests your lower body force production (vertical countermovement jump), reactive strength (drop jump), linear speed (30m sprint), and aerobic fitness (maximum aerobic speed test).

The tool then creates 4-week targets and generates exercise recommendations.

Helpful FREE Content!

Link and QR Code on the last page.

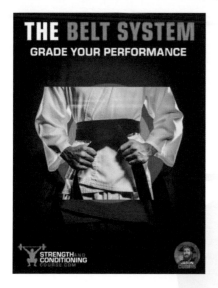

The Belt System was designed as a FUN way for clients and athletes to set targets. However, we were amazed at how popular it became - the increases in motivation have been huge!

There are 5 disciplines, 8 tests per discipline, and 8 coloured belts up for grabs!

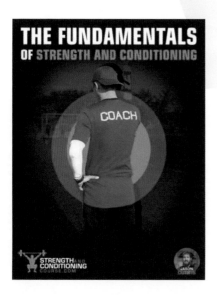

This download takes a look at what it takes to become a strength and conditioning coach and our unique BIG 8 model.

Programming & Periodization / Warming Up / Strength Training / Ballistic Training / Olympic Weightlifting / Plyometrics / Speed & Agility / Metabolic Conditioning.

Our Courses

Link and QR Code on the last page.

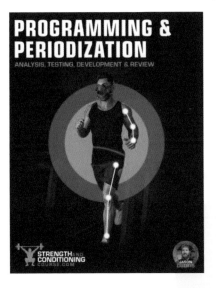

This course details each fundamental step to creating the optimal plan:

The Needs Analysis of both the Sport and Athlete. Testing of the Athlete. Analysis of the Results. Development of the Periodized Plan. Programming of Sessions. Evaluations and Modifications.

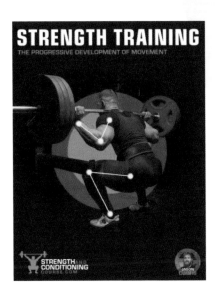

The development of strength is the foundation of physical performance because, before all else, you need the strength in your structures to support the fundamental movements that you carry out each day.

This HUGE course consists of 240+ narrated slides and 4+ hours of video tutorials for over 100 exercises.

Our Courses

Link and QR Code on the last page.

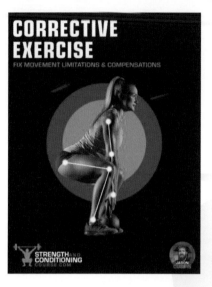

This course is designed for fitness professionals and enthusiasts who want to gain an in-depth understanding of how to fix technique faults and compensation patterns caused by mobility restrictions, muscular imbalances, and asymmetries.

Maximize performance and minimize your risk of injury.

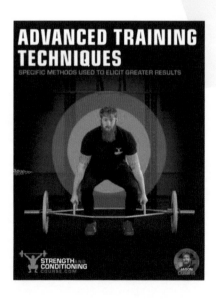

If you want to learn how to smash plateaus and take your training to the next level, this short course is perfect for you.

This course includes over 50 advanced training techniques, many with numerous variations.

A must for those that want greater results!

Check out all our content by using the link below or scanning the QR code:

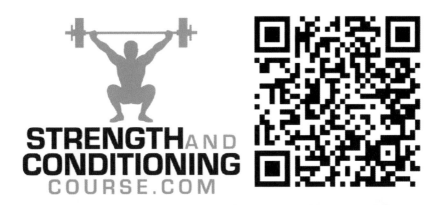

https://courses.strengthandconditioningcourse.com

Purchase any of my other books here:

https://jasoncurtis.org

Scan the QR Code/use the link below to get access to all of my FREE content:

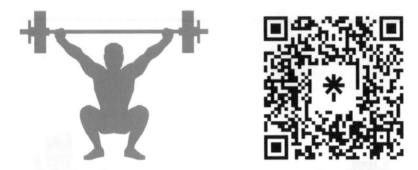

https://linktr.ee/sccacademy

Be social and follow us on our Instagram:

https://instagram.com/strengthandconditioningcourse